£8-95

# AIDS TO CLINICAL EXAMINATI

G000240886

For Churchill Livingstone

*Publisher:* Laurence Hunter
*Editorial Co-ordination:* Editorial Resources Unit
  *Copy Editor:* Delia Malim-Robinson
*Production:* I. Macaulay Hunter
*Design:* Design Resources Unit
*Sales Promotion Executive:* Marion Pollock

# AIDS TO CLINICAL EXAMINATION

## Peter C. Hayes

BMSc (Hons) MB ChB (Hons) MRCP MD
Senior Lecturer and Honorary Consultant Physician,
Department of Medicine,
Royal Infirmary, Edinburgh

## Ronald S. MacWalter

BMSc (Hons) MB ChB (Hons) MRCP
Consultant Physician in Medicine for the Elderly
and Honorary Senior Lecturer,
Section of Ageing and Health,
Department of Medicine,
Ninewells Hospital and Medical School,
Dundee

SECOND EDITION

CHURCHILL LIVINGSTONE
EDINBURGH LONDON MADRID MELBOURNE NEW YORK AND TOKYO 1992

CHURCHILL LIVINGSTONE
Medical Division of Longman Group UK Limited

Distributed in the United States of America by
Churchill Livingstone Inc., 650 Avenue of the
Americas, New York, N.Y. 10011, and by
associated companies, branches and
representatives throughout the world.

First edition 1986
Second edition 1992

ISBN 0-443-04572-0

**British Library Cataloguing in Publication Data**
A catalogue record for this book is available from
the British Library.

**Library of Congress Cataloging in Publication Data**
Hayes, Peter C.
    Aids to clinical examination/Peter C. Hayes,
Ronald S. MacWalter. — 2nd ed.
        p.  cm.
    Includes index.
    ISBN 0-443-04572-0
    1. Physical diagnosis—Outlines, syllabi, etc.
I. MacWalter, Ronald S.  II. Title.
    [DNLM: 1. Diagnosis—outlines. 2. Physical
Examination—outlines. WB 18 H418a]
RC76.H34 1992
616.07'5—dc20
DNLM/DLC
for Library of Congress                    91-29751
                                                CIP

Produced by Longman Singapore Publishers Pte Ltd
Printed in Singapore

# PREFACE TO THE SECOND EDITION

The intention of this book is to fill a gap in examination preparation. Examinations of clinical skill, like written examinations, require revision and this book is designed to help with this. It is written to replace the cards so often prepared by the student about how to examine a system or patient under examination settings. It is principally written to help students preparing for undergraduate 'final examinations' and those studying for such postgraduate diplomas as the MRCP. However, we hope it will prove useful to students studying for any form of clinical examination.

The structure of the book is such that the headings down the left-hand side of the page can act as an aide-mémoire or checklist of things to look for, whilst the accompanying notes provide useful tips and explanations. This format also allows candidates to add notes to the text. It is realised that examinations of clinical skill are conducted under artificial circumstances and that certain procedures normally part of clinical practice, such as the rectal examination, will not be required. They are, however, included in the text for completeness. To keep each chapter as a relatively separate entity, a certain amount of repetition was necessary to avoid excessive cross-referencing.

We are aware that this form of presentation lends itself better to certain systems than others, but have stuck to the same format throughout in the belief that it will encourage systematic examination.

Clinical practice evolves to meet changing needs and priorities. Accordingly, new chapters on stroke, confused patients, AIDS, and examination technique have been added. The other chapters have been modified to take account of developments. The book has retained its pocket-size appeal.

In medicine it is important to prepare thoroughly before any examination, but this ethic should continue when dealing with any patient. This book can aid in preparation for examination and also in the audit of daily clinical performance.

We hope this new edition will be appreciated by as many readers as the first.

Edinburgh and Dundee                                         P.C.H.
1992                                                         R.S.M.

We would like to acknowledge the patience and help of our wives, Sharon and Sheila.

# CONTENTS

Notes for clinical examinations 1

1. Hands 3

2. Face 10

3. Eyes 18

4. Cranial nerves 26

5. Neck 30

6. Cardiovascular system 37

7. Respiratory system 50

8. Abdomen 56

9. Legs 66

10. Anaemia 73

11. Polycythaemia 78

12. Cyanosis 81

13. Jaundice 85

14. Uraemia 90

15. Diabetes mellitus 95

16. Thyrotoxicosis 99

17. Hypertension 102

18. Stroke 107

19. Ataxia 114

20. Confused patient 120

21. Arthritis 124

22. HIV infection 132

Index 135

# NOTES FOR CLINICAL EXAMINATIONS

Sitting clinical examinations is something of an art where the unpractised, even if knowledgeable, can come unstuck, whilst the well-trained, even if of only average ability, can impress. Below are a few hints about taking clinical examinations:

1. Turn up smartly dressed, wearing nothing provocative. This may seem to be conforming, but examiners (and patients) expect it.

2. Practise repeatedly subjects likely to be asked (e.g. examination of the chest, heart and abdomen) until they become second nature. This is far more worthwhile than spending hours practising things less likely to appear (e.g. eliciting cerebellar signs, testing all cranial nerves).

3. Similarly, know what hypertensive and diabetic fundi look like and how to describe them.

4. Practise verbal presentation of the cases. Many candidates examine the patient well and then appear very hesitant when it comes to describing their findings.

5. While it is quite sensible to have a familiar ophthalmoscope with you, do carry it discreetly. Do not carry around armfuls of tendon hammers and other implements. This is tempting fate, and most candidates would prefer to avoid being asked to examine a neurological case. It is also likely that you will leave some of the equipment at a bedside and have to go back, disrupting the exam.

6. Remember your stethoscope; there is always someone who forgets and it creates a very poor impression.

7. When asked for the diagnosis, if you know it, give it. Do not vacillate, giving a large list of unlikely differential diagnoses.

8. Do not mention rare diseases unnecessarily just to impress, especially if you know little about them. You are tempting the examiner to ask 'Tell me what you know about that condition?'

9. Remember that most people who fail the examination do so for getting the basics wrong, not because they misinterpreted some

obscure sign. Ignore the apocryphal stories about people who failed for not identifying Kayser–Fleischer rings. (They probably were not these anyway.)

10. Do not take beta blockers to reduce stress, and try to avoid mopping your brow in public.

# 1. HANDS

| | |
|---|---|
| **INSPECTION** | Hands frequently provide clues of underlying disease and should be closely inspected. They are a logical starting point for examination in all patients. |
| **Size** | The overall size should be noted and interpreted in the context of body size. Enlargement may be due to acromegaly (when they are described as spade-like), obesity, hypothyroidism, primary amyloidosis and manual work. Unilateral enlargement may be due to oedema such as occurs in venous or lymphatic obstruction and disuse (e.g. hemiplegia). |
| **Involuntary Movement** | Involuntary movement may be important diagnostically. Tremors may be resting, postural or action. |
| *Coarse tremor* | A coarse tremor at rest is seen in Parkinson's disease and is characteristically 'pill-rolling'. |
| *Physiological tremor* | The physiological tremor is a fine postural tremor, and an exaggerated form may be seen in anxiety states, hyperthyroidism and alcoholism. |
| *Benign essential tremor* | The benign essential tremor occurs more commonly in the elderly, may be familial and may be abolished by alcohol. It is a postural tremor. |
| *Intention tremor* | This action tremor occurs with voluntary movement and worsens as the end-point in the movement is reached: it is tested for in the 'finger-nose' test and is a feature of cerebellar disease (Ch. 19). |
| *Asterixis* | Asterixis is a flapping tremor, elicited by dorsiflexion of hands with the arms outstretched. It is seen in hepatic failure, uraemia, hypercapnia, |

congestive cardiac failure and Wernicke's encephalopathy.

*Fasciculation*

Fasciculation, the spontaneous firing of individual motor units, may be seen involving the small muscles of the hand. Although it occurs in normal subjects, lower motor neurone damage and particularly motor neurone disease should be considered, especially if there is associated muscle wasting.

## Palms

*Erythema*

Palmar erythema is seen in chronic liver disease, rheumatoid arthritis, thyrotoxicosis and pregnancy.

*Hyperkeratosis (rare)*

Hyperkeratosis of the palms is seen in tylosis (a rare familial disorder associated with increased risk of oesophageal carcinoma).

*Dupuytren's contracture*

Dupuytren's contracture (palmar fascia fibrosis) occurs primarily in males and may have a higher incidence in patients with alcoholic liver disease, although this is disputed. It is also reputed to occur in association with manual work, insulin-dependent diabetes mellitus and epilepsy. It is common in otherwise normal subjects and may be familial. It typically affects the ring finger first and is usually bilateral, although frequently asymmetrical.

*Skin creases*

Skin creases are pale in anaemia, darkly pigmented in Addison's disease, and yellow in carotinaemia.

*Cyanosis*

Fingers, and nail beds in particular, are blue in cyanosis. If the hand is warm and cyanosed, central cyanosis exists (see Ch. 12).

*Muscle wasting*

Thenar eminence atrophy is seen in median nerve lesions (e.g. carpal tunnel syndrome) while hypothenar eminence wasting occurs with ulnar nerve lesions. Atrophy of the small muscles of the hand is seen in $T_1$ root lesions, motor neurone disease, syringomyelia, cord compression, cervical rib, Klumpke's paralysis, cervical spondylosis, neurofibromata, injuries to brachial, ulnar or median nerves, arthritis (especially rheumatoid) and generalised cachexia.

| | |
|---|---|
| *Rashes* | Rashes are unusual in the palms of the hands but occur in secondary syphilis, pompholyx and pustular psoriasis. |

**Nails**

| | |
|---|---|
| *Clubbing* | Finger clubbing is a hallmark of many diseases and an important physical sign. Five stages of clubbing are recognised: |

1. Increased nail bed fluctuation (examine with index fingers of each hand over the nail bed of the finger to be examined with the thumbs underneath).
2. Loss of nail bed angle (normally 140°).
3. Increased curvature of long axis of nail.
4. Soft tissue swelling at the end of the finger which when marked produces a drum-stick appearance.
5. Hypertrophic pulmonary osteoarthropathy may develop and is recognised by painful wrists and periosteal elevation demonstrated radiologically.

Causes of clubbing can be divided into respiratory, which include bronchiectasis, bronchial carcinoma, mesothelioma, asbestosis, empyema, and fibrosing alveolitis, and non-respiratory, which include infective endocarditis, cyanotic congenital cardiac disease, atrial myxoma, hepatic cirrhosis, Crohn's disease, panproctocolitis, coeliac disease, brachial arteriovenous fistula (causes unilateral clubbing), thyrotoxicosis, dysproteinaemia (especially alpha-chain disease), pyelonephritis, syphilis, pregnancy and congenital.

| | |
|---|---|
| *Pseudo-clubbing* | Resorption of the terminal phalanges may be seen in hyperparathyroidism, giving an appearance similar to finger clubbing — pseudo-clubbing. |
| *Koilonychia* | Koilonychia (spoon-shaped deformity) is said to be commoner in iron deficiency, although specificity is poor. |
| *Leukonychia* | Leukonychia (white discoloration) is seen in hypoalbuminaemia with or without liver disease. |
| *Lindsay's nails* | Lindsay's nails are half white/half brown nails found in patients with chronic renal disease. |

| | |
|---|---|
| *Terry's nails* | Opaque white nails often with pink distal zone may occur in cirrhosis. |
| *Splinter haemorrhages* | Longitudinal splinter haemorrhages occur in infective endocarditis and after nail trauma. Transverse splinter haemorrhages are seen in trichinosis. |
| *Onycholysis* | Onycholysis, where the nail becomes detached distally from its plate, occurs in thyrotoxicosis, eczema, psoriasis and fungal infections. |
| *Beau's lines* | In severe illnesses, transverse indentations (Beau's lines) may occur. Longitudinal ridges are usually due to trauma. |
| *Pitting* | As well as causing onycholysis, psoriasis may produce pitting of nails. This is often associated with psoriatic arthropathy of affected fingers. |
| *Nail bed infarcts* | Nail bed infarcts indicate a vasculitic process and are seen particularly in systemic lupus erythematosus and rheumatoid disease. |
| *Telangiectasia of nail folds* | In dermatomyositis and systemic lupus erythematosus, telangiectasia of nail folds may be seen. |
| *Absent nails* | Congenital absence of nails occurs and may be associated with other congenital abnormalities such as absent or rudimentary patellae. Nails may also be absent because of previous trauma or nail bed infections. |
| *Yellow nail syndrome* | The triad of yellow nails, lymphatic oedema of lower limbs and sterile pleural effusion, is known as the yellow nail syndrome (cause unknown). |
| *Blue lunulae* | The lunulae may be coloured blue in Wilson's disease (hepatolenticular degeneration) due to increased copper deposition. |
| *Tar staining* | Heavily tar-stained nails and fingers may reflect more the habit of smoking a cigarette down to the butt than the number smoked per day! |
| *Periungual fibroma (rare)* | Hypertrophic nodules around nails — periungual fibroma — which may look like viral warts, are associated with tuberous sclerosis. |
| *Fungal infections* | Chronic fungal infections produce atrophic nails as in familial hypoparathyroidism. |

## Other Lesions

| | |
|---|---|
| *Scabies* | Red excoriated lesions, especially at the finger web area, are seen with scabies infections; the burrows are characteristic. |

**Joints** (see Ch. 21)

| | |
|---|---|
| *Rheumatoid arthritis* | Rheumatoid arthritis, the symmetrical, proximal arthropathy, results in synovitis of the metacarpophalangeal joints, with filling of the hollow between metacarpal heads when the fingers are flexed and synovial swelling of extensor tendon sheaths. Tendon tears produce 'swan neck' and 'boutonnière' deformities. Swelling of the proximal interphalangeal joints produces spindle-shaped deformity (Haygarth nodes). Marked deformity may exist at the wrists. Carpal tunnel syndrome may coexist and is due to synovial hypertrophy. Check for rheumatoid nodules at the elbow and for vasculitis in the skin. |
| *Osteoarthrosis* | Heberden's nodes occur at the distal interphalangeal joints in familial generalised osteoarthrosis. Bouchard's nodes occur at proximal interphalangeal joints. The 'square hand' deformity is due to involvement of the thumb carpometacarpal joint. A gross but painless osteoarthrosis (Charcot's joint) may be seen in the hand in leprosy, and wrist (elbow and shoulder) in syringomyelia. |
| *Gout* | Gout produces an asymmetrical pattern of arthritis with tophaceous swelling in relation to joints. The helix of the ear should also be inspected for tophi. |
| *Psoriatic arthropathy* | Look for the typical rash and nail changes. Arthritis mutilans with telescoping fingers is characteristic but can also be seen in rheumatoid arthritis and other connective tissue disorders. |
| *Pseudohypoparathyroidism* | The hand in pseudohypoparathyroidism has a characteristic appearance with shortening of the fourth metacarpal which is made more readily apparent when a fist is made. |

---

| | |
|---|---|
| **PALPATION** | Before palpating the hands ascertain whether there are any painful or tender lesions as it is important not to add to the patient's discomfort. |
| *Osler's nodes (rare)* | The finger pulps should be palpated to identify Osler's nodes which are exquisitely tender |

| | nodules that occur rarely in infective endocarditis. |
|---|---|
| *Joint tenderness* | All joints should be tested for tenderness either individually or with a squeeze test examining rows of joints, the examiner being careful not to hurt the patient. |
| *Hypertrophic pulmonary arthropathy* | Tenderness around the wrist associated with finger clubbing occurs in hypertrophic pulmonary osteoarthropathy. |
| **Passive Joint Movement** | All joints should be put through a full range of passive movement, care being taken not to cause pain. Also note whether joint crepitus occurs with movement. |
| **Active Joint Movement and Power** | Assess grip strength and power of extension at wrist and fingers and small muscles of hand. |
| *Median nerve* | The median nerve supplies the lateral two lumbricals, opponens pollicis, abductor pollicis brevis and flexor pollicis brevis (mnemonic LOAF). The abductor pollicis brevis is tested by straight raising of the thumb vertically with the back of hand flat on a table. |
| *Ulnar nerve* | The ulnar nerve supplies all the other small muscles of the hand. An ulnar nerve lesion below the elbow produces clawing of fourth and fifth fingers. Test for joint hyper-extension at the metacarpophalangeal joints and assess abduction and adduction of the fingers. Weakness of adductor pollicis produces Froment's sign which is detected by applying traction to a sheet of paper held between the thumb and clenched fist of both the patient's hands. Weakness of the adductor pollicis causes flexion of the distal phalanx of the thumb (Froment's sign). |
| *Radial nerve* | A radial nerve lesion causes wrist drop with weakness of triceps, extensor carpiradialis, extensor digitalis and extensor pollicis longus. Weakness of the extensors also produces considerable weakness of flexors as the antagonists which are necessary for stability are removed. |
| **Sensation** | Abnormal sensation may be demonstrable in the hands. Three main patterns of sensory loss are |

recognised — firstly involving segmental distribution, secondly involving peripheral nerves, and thirdly involving a glove and stocking distribution as in a peripheral neuropathy (Fig. 1.1).

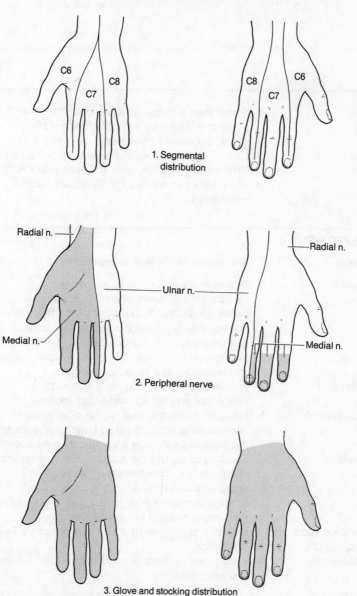

1. Segmental distribution

2. Peripheral nerve

3. Glove and stocking distribution

**Fig. 1.1** Innervation abnormalities of the hand.

# 2. FACE

Sometimes a glance at a particular face may suggest a diagnosis and confirmatory signs should be sought elsewhere (see Table 2.1). Careful systematic examination may be required. When examining the face, the eyes (see Ch. 3) and cranial nerves (see Ch. 4) should also be considered.

## INSPECTION

**Shape**

The shape of the face is important.

*Cheeks*

Drawn-in cheeks are seen in cachexia (e.g. cancer, chronic heart failure), thyrotoxicosis and partial lipodystrophy. Fullness of the face may be due to obesity, Cushing's syndrome, acute glomerulonephritis, parotid swelling (as in mumps, parotitis, parotid tumours, sarcoidosis), and superior vena caval obstruction.

*Bossing*

Frontal bossing may be seen in rickets, congenital syphilis and sickle cell anaemia.

*Skull enlargement*

Enlargement of the vault of the skull lends a characteristic appearance to Paget's disease of the skull (cranial nerve entrapments may occur).

*Swelling*

Swelling of part of the face, with erythema and a sharp margin of demarcation, is seen in erysipelas while angioneurotic oedema and contact dermatitis (e.g. to drugs or eye make-up) may cause marked localised facial swelling.

*Marfan's syndrome*

Marfan's syndrome might be suggested by facial elongation.

*Acromegaly*

In acromegaly there is coarsening of the features and prognathia.

**Colour**

The colour of the complexion is worth noting.

**Table 2.1**   Typical facial appearances in some conditions with certain associated signs

| Condition | Facial Appearance | Other Signs |
|---|---|---|
| Down's syndrome | Round face<br>Prominent epicanthic folds<br>Low nasal bridge<br>Large fissured tongue | Simian crease<br>Incurved little finger<br>Mental retardation |
| Hypothyroidism | Puffy face<br>Coarsened features<br>Coarse dry hair | Hoarse voice<br>Bradycardia<br>Delayed tendon jerk relaxation |
| Hyperthyroidism | Anxious, staring (eye signs)<br>Sweating | Tachycardia<br>Tremor (clubbing, pretibial myxoedema) |
| Cushing's syndrome | Round moon face<br>Plethora | 'Lemon on sticks' appearance<br>Buffalo hump, striae (hirsutism) |
| Addison's disease | Hyperpigmented | Pigmented palmar crease and buccal mucosa |
| Acromegaly | Coarse features<br>Prominent jaw, nose, lower lip | Large hands and feet (bitemporal hemianopia) |
| Paget's disease | Increased skull size<br>Platybasia (cranial nerve palsies) | |
| Parkinson's disease | Expressionless face<br>Excess sebum secretion<br>Drooling of saliva | Tremor<br>Extra pyramidal rigidity<br>Akinesia |
| Dystrophia myotonica | Frontal baldness<br>Wasted facial muscles<br>Transverse smile | Sternomastoid wasting<br>Cataract |
| Facial palsy (LMN) (Bell's palsy) | Facial weakness on affected side<br>Affects forehead muscles | Cannot close eye (Bell's sign) |
| Scleroderma (systemic sclerosis) | Tightening of skin over nose and around mouth<br>Telangiectases | Sclerodactyly, Raynaud's (calcinosis — CRST) |

| | |
|---|---|
| *Pallor* | Pallor is seen in anaemia, vasoconstriction, malnutrition and panhypopituitarism. |
| *Vitiligo* | Localised depigmentation as vitiligo may suggest an underlying autoimmune disorder or be idiopathic. Total failure of pigment production is |
| *Albinism* | seen in albinism. |
| *Pigmentation* | Melanin pigmentation may indicate racial origin. Increased pigmentation is seen in Addison's |

|                      | disease, haemochromatosis, primary biliary cirrhosis and renal failure. |
|----------------------|--------------------------------------------------------------------------|
| *Chloasma*           | Chloasma — patchy pigmentation over forehead and around eyes — may occur in pregnancy or be due to the oral contraceptive pill. |
| *Pigmented lesions*  | Pigmented lesions may be benign, such as freckles, simple naevi and seborrhoeic keratoses (greasy, warty lesions associated with increasing age), or malignant, such as malignant melanoma, which may bleed or ulcerate. |
| *Jaundice*           | Jaundice (see Ch. 13). |
| *Plethora*           | Plethora may reflect outdoor occupation, polycythaemia or carcinoid syndrome. A malar flush may be seen in mitral stenosis and Cushing's syndrome, whilst a 'peaches and cream' appearance is seen in hypothyroidism (excess carotene gives yellowish tinge). The butterfly rash of discoid and systemic lupus erythematosus must be distinguished from facial plethora. Easy flushing is seen in acne rosacea and the carcinoid syndrome, while generalised erythema affecting the face (l'homme rouge) may be associated with an underlying lymphoproliferative disease. |

**Emotional State**  The emotional state should be noted.

| *Agitation*          | Agitation is seen in anxiety, mania and |
| *Apathy*             | hyperthyroidism, while apathy is typical of depression and hypothyroidism. |
| *Lack of expression* | Lack of facial expression due to poverty of movement is seen in parkinsonism. |
| *Emotional lability* | Emotional lability may complicate cerebrovascular accidents, especially when pseudobulbar palsy is also present. This feature may mask an underlying depression. |
| *Euphoria*           | Frank euphoria is sometimes seen in multiple |
| *Cheerfulness*       | sclerosis, while cheerfulness in the face of apparent adversity may be a sign of hysteria. |

**Hair**

| *Frontal balding*    | Frontal balding is a characteristic feature of dystrophia myotonica but is common in males. |
| *Alopecia*           | Patchy hair loss (alopecia) is seen in alopecia areata (characteristic 'exclamation-mark' hairs — normal width at the tip and narrow at the base — are found at the margins during the active phase), excessive hair-pulling (trichotillomania), |

|  | secondary to cytotoxic drugs, and scarring alopecia secondary to systemic lupus erythematosus, scleroderma, lichen planus, and severe fungal and bacterial infections. |
|---|---|
| *Thinning* | Generalised thinning of the hair may be seen in Cushing's syndrome and hypothyroidism. |
| *Coarsening* | Coarsening of the hair is also a feature of hypothyroidism. |
| *Hirsutism* | Hirsutism may be seen with adrenal lesions (adrenal tumours, Cushing's syndrome and congenital adrenal hyperplasia), be drug induced (e.g. minoxidil), or associated with ovarian lesions (arrhenoblastoma and polycystic ovaries). More commonly, however, it is familial, racial or idiopathic. |
| *Lack of facial hair* | Lack of facial hair is seen in hypogonadism, whilst regression of facial hair may occur in hypopituitarism. |

**Skin**

| **Skin** | Examination of the facial skin may show lesions of a primary skin disorder or those associated with an underlying disease. |
|---|---|
| *Facial rashes* | Facial rashes are common and must be identified. |
| *SLE* | In systemic lupus erythematosus a scaly erythematous rash with typical batswing distribution over cheeks and bridge of nose occurs with scarring and atrophy. |
| *Dermatomyositis* | A heliotrope rash, especially over the eyelids, temples and cheeks (but also on the knuckles) may occur in dermatomyositis. |
| *Acne rosacea* | Acne rosacea occurs typically over the cheeks and nose and is erythematous with pustules and telangiectasia. |
| *Carcinoid* | Flushing is a feature of carcinoid syndrome; this may progress to persistent redness. |
| *Perioral dermatitis* | An erythematous papular eruption around the mouth, perioral dermatitis, may be seen in young women. |
| *Acne vulgaris* | Acne vulgaris with its characteristic folliculitis, pustule formation, comedones and excess sebum secretion, affects the face, neck, shoulders and chest in adolescence, but is also associated with the oral contraceptive pill, Cushing's syndrome and phenytoin use. |
| *Seborrhoeic dermatitis* | Seborrhoeic dermatitis is common and affects flexural areas, nasolabial fold and causes scaliness of the eyebrows. |

| | |
|---|---|
| *Atopic eczema* | Atopic eczema is usually intensely pruritic and scratch marks may be seen as well as the exuding patches involving the cheeks, ears and scalp, which may progress to lichenification. |
| *Psoriasis* | Psoriatic plaques rarely occur on the face but are sometimes seen around the scalp margin, eyes, nose and ears. |
| *Drugs* | Drugs can cause any type of rash, although erythematous maculopapular types are common. |
| *Stevens–Johnson syndrome* | Stevens–Johnson syndrome, cutaneous erythema multiforme with ulceration of mucous membranes, can be associated with drug use (e.g. penicillin and sulphonamides), but may also occur in bacterial and viral infections. |
| *Light exposure* *SLE* *Polymorphic light eruption* *Porphyrias (rare)* | Rashes in light-exposed areas are seen in systemic lupus erythematosus, polymorphic light eruption (rashes of various types), and the porphyrias. In porphyria cutanea tarda and porphyria variegata, bullous eruptions may be noted; in erythropoietic protoporphyria pock-marking is seen, while in erythropoietic porphyria, bullous destructive lesions are noted together with deformed and reddened teeth. |
| *Pemphigus* | Pemphigus may affect the face and mouth. The bullous lesions strip on pressure (Nikolski's sign), heal without scarring and are intra-epidermal, |
| *Pemphigoid* | while pemphigoid has tense, large blisters which are sub-epidermal and may be associated with underlying malignancy. |
| *Dermatitis herpetiformis* | Dermatitis herpetiformis — clusters of small, pruritic blisters (also on shoulders, lumbosacral area, elbows and knees) — may be associated with coeliac disease. |
| *Blisters* | Blisters can be due to heat-induced trauma and drug overdose (e.g. phenobarbitone) where pressure areas tend to be affected. |
| *Toxic epidermal necrolysis* | Toxic epidermal necrolysis, due to staphylococcal infection, is characterised by large blisters and crusting. |
| *Furuncles* | Furuncles (boils) are due to staphylococcal infection of hair follicles. They occur more frequently in diabetics. When a cluster of adjacent follicles is involved this larger lesion is |
| *Carbuncle* | called a carbuncle. |
| *Impetigo* | Impetigo is a spreading infection of the epidermis common in children. |

| | |
|---|---|
| *Syphilis* | A primary syphilitic chancre may rarely be seen on the lips or in the mouth, while snail track ulcers of the mouth and a maculopapular rash are seen in secondary syphilis. |
| *Lupus vulgaris* | Lupus vulgaris, cutaneous tuberculosis, produces erythematous, hypertrophic, ulcerative lesions which may erode and scar. A glass-slide applied over the lesion produces an 'apple-jelly' appearance. |
| *Lupus pernio* | Lupus pernio are raised bluish-red plaques found particularly over the nose in sarcoidosis. |
| *Leprosy* | In lepromatous leprosy, nodular granulomatous lesions on the face are seen (leonine facies) while in tuberculoid leprosy, lesions may be hypopigmented and anaesthetic. |
| *Ringworm* | Ringworm may affect the scalp and face. On the scalp affected hairs are broken off leaving the scalp scaled and inflamed. Similar lesions may be seen on the face. |
| *Candida* | Candida albicans infection may cause angular cheilitis (associated with poorly-fitting dentures and vitamin deficiency), and white adherent plaques in the mouth (thrush). |
| *Pityriasis versicolor* | Pityriasis versicolor, due to the microorganism *Malassezia furfur*, produces a scaly rash with areas of depigmentation. |
| *Molluscum contagiosum* *Warts* | Molluscum contagiosum (cream-coloured umbilicated globular nodules) and warts are caused by viral infections. |
| *Herpes simplex* | Herpes simplex, the familiar vesicular crusting cold sores, reflects secondary recrudescence of dormant infection often associated with debility or pneumonia and may be extensive in immunosuppressed patients. The primary infection itself may be severe with stomatitis and pharyngitis. |
| *Herpes zoster* *Ramsay–Hunt syndrome* | The maculovesicular rash of herpes zoster (shingles) may affect part of the distribution of the trigeminal nerve with pain and parasthesiae and, rarely, motor disturbance. The Ramsay–Hunt syndrome consists of facial palsy due to herpes zoster infection of geniculate ganglion associated with skin lesions in the external auditory meatus. |
| *Spider naevi* | Spider naevi may be seen in liver disease, pregnancy and rheumatoid arthritis (see Ch. 8). |

| | |
|---|---|
| *Telangiectases* | Telangiectases are seen in systemic sclerosis and hereditary haemorrhagic telangiectasia. |
| *Cavernous haemangiomas* *Capillary haemangiomas* | Cavernous haemangiomas (strawberry naevi) are nodular and resolve spontaneously while capillary haemangiomas (port-wine stain) remain and may be associated with a meningeal haemangioma (Sturge–Weber syndrome). |
| *Adenoma sebaceum* | Adenoma sebaceum are hamartomas of connective tissue and should suggest tuberous sclerosis. |
| *Lentigines* | Pigmented lentigines affecting the face and lips occur in Peutz–Jegher's syndrome. |
| *Lentigo maligna* | Lentigo maligna or Hutchison's melanotic freckle, a solitary flat dark lesion which spreads slowly, is seen in the elderly and may progress to malignant melanoma. |
| *Malignant melanoma* | Malignant melanomas may be pigmented, nodular, ulcerating lesions which may bleed or crust. They may, however, be entirely amelanotic. |
| *Solar keratoses* | Solar keratoses, small irregular scaly warty plaques, are seen in fair-skinned people exposed to excessive sunlight. |
| *Basal cell carcinoma* | Basal cell carcinomas (rodent ulcers) usually have a rolled edge and destructive centre and are associated with excess sunlight exposure. They may be seen as part of Gorlin's syndrome (with palmar pits, mandibular cysts and central nervous system tumours). |
| *Kerato-acanthomas* *Squamous cell carcinoma* | Kerato-acanthomas are rapidly growing warty lesions with a central horny plug seen on light-exposed areas and which are sometimes difficult to distinguish from squamous cell carcinomas. |
| *Metastases* | Deposits of metastatic carcinoma are sometimes found on the face or scalp. |
| *Xanthelasma* | See Chapter 3. |

**Nose**

| | |
|---|---|
| *Rhinophyma* | Inspection of the nose may reveal rhinophyma, where the nose is enlarged, red and bulbous in the late stages of acne rosacea. |
| *Destruction of nasal cartilage* | Destruction of nasal cartilage is seen in tertiary syphilis, Wegner's granulomatosis, lupus vulgaris, leprosy and chronic relapsing |

polychondritis while deformity is often simply due to old trauma.

*Discharge*  A purulent discharge is seen in chronic sinusitis (consider Kartagener's syndrome) whilst a serous discharge occurs in hay fever and coryza.

**Ears**

*Gouty tophi*  White nodules on the helix of the ear, gouty tophi, are due to deposition of sodium biurate

*Darwin's tubercle*  crystals (do not confuse with Darwin's tubercle, a normal variant.) Dusky pigmentation of the

*Alkaptonuria*  cartilage of the ear is seen in alkaptonuria.

*Hairy pinna*  Hairy pinnae are sometimes inherited as a Y-linked trait.

---

## PALPATION

*Temporal arteries*  The temporal arteries may be tender or non-pulsatile in temporal arteritis.

*Swellings*  Any swelling should be palpated and its nature, size and associated lymphadenopathy (if any) identified (see Ch. 5).

*Eyes*  See Chapter 3.

---

## PERCUSSION

Percussion of the face and head has limited application.

*Chvostek's sign*  Tapping over the facial nerve anterior to the ear in hypocalcaemia may produce twitching of facial muscles, especially the upper lip (Chvostek's sign).

*Percussive auscultation*  Percussive auscultation of the skull, where the forehead is percussed whilst different areas of the skull are listened to, has been proposed as a useful method of detecting extradural haematomas. In children with raised intracranial pressure, a 'cracked pot' note occurs on percussion.

---

## AUSCULTATION

Auscultation over the eyeball and head may disclose bruits due to arterio-venous malformations.

# 3. EYES

---

## INSPECTION

### General

**Proptosis**

The eyes should be inspected from the front, sides and from above to avoid missing mild proptosis. From the front particular attention should be paid to apparent size and symmetry. Slight differences in the palpebral fissure should be looked for and an assessment made as to whether lid retraction in one eye or ptosis of the other is responsible for the asymmetry.

**Lid retraction**

Lid retraction is usually bilateral and is recognised when a rim of sclera is present above the iris. Causes of lid retraction include thyrotoxicosis and situations associated with sympathetic overactivity, e.g. left ventricular failure, phaeochromocytoma.

**Ptosis**

Causes of ptosis can be divided into muscular, such as myasthenia gravis and dystrophia myotonica, or neurological, such as Horner's syndrome. A complete ptosis accompanies third cranial nerve palsy.

**Lid lag**

Lid lag is frequently associated with lid retraction and should be looked for by asking the patient to stare at the examiner's finger as it is moved slowly up and down. The upper eyelid is delayed in following the downward movement of the eye. This is a useful confirmatory sign when thyrotoxicosis is suspected.

**Exophthalmos**

Exophthalmos is recognised when a rim of sclera is seen both above and below the iris. An exophthalmometer should be used to measure the degree of exophthalmos. It may be unilateral as with periorbital neoplasms or infections and carotico-cavernous sinus fistulae. Although cavernous sinus thrombosis may cause bilateral exophthalmos, the commonest cause by far is thyrotoxicosis. It should be remembered that there may be marked asymmetry in the severity of exophthalmos in each eye and that there may be no other signs of thyroid overactivity present.

*Glass eye*  It is sometimes quite difficult to detect a glass eye!

## Eyelids

*Blinking*  The frequency of blinking should be noted. In parkinsonism and in some blind patients it may be infrequent.

*Ectropion*  Ectropion, or eversion of the lower lid, is common in the elderly, and may be associated with chronic facial palsy.

*Entropion*  Entropion or inversion of the lower lid complicates severe blepharitis and trachoma.

*Hordeolum*  Infection around an eyelash, a hordeolum or sty, is common; the other swelling of the lid which

*Chalazion*  involves the meibomian glands is the chalazion. Inflammation of the lacrimal glands,

*Dacryoadenitis*  dacryoadenitis, produces swelling in the upper outer aspect of the eyelid. Bilateral dacryoadenitis occurs with sarcoidosis, syphilis, tuberculosis and leukaemia.

*Periorbital and lid oedema*  Periorbital and lid oedema may occur in association with local infection or be a feature of hypothyroidism, cardiac failure and nephrotic syndrome.

*Xanthelasma*  Xanthelasma, cholesterol deposits in the eyelids, occur with chronic obstructive jaundice, diabetes mellitus, myxoedema, nephrotic syndrome and familial hypercholesterolaemia. Signs elsewhere may aid in the diagnosis.

## Conjunctiva

*Conjunctivitis*  Injection of the conjunctival blood vessels reflects conjunctival inflammation. It is usually bilateral and causes include bacterial and viral infection, foreign body (unilateral), allergies, sarcoidosis, tuberculosis and Stevens–Johnson syndrome.

*Chemosis*  Chemosis, oedema of the conjunctiva, occurs in severe infections, cavernous sinus thrombosis, retro-orbital tumours and with severe exophthalmos.

*Pallor*  Conjunctival pallor may indicate anaemia.

## Sclera

| | |
|---|---|
| *Jaundice* | The sclera should be examined for jaundice. |
| *Blue discoloration* | Blue discoloration of the sclera occurs in osteogenesis imperfecta. In the elderly, choroidal pigment may be visible through the sclera. |
| *Episcleritis* | Occasionally systemic disorders such as rheumatoid disease and sarcoidosis may cause episcleritis. In rheumatoid disease this may proceed to ulceration and perforation of the sclera (scleromalacia perforans). |

## Iris

| | |
|---|---|
| | The iris should be inspected with a bright light at the same time as testing the pupillary reflexes. |
| *Brushfield spots* | Brushfield spots — small white areas — are seen in Down's syndrome. |
| *Iritis* | Iritis is characterised by injection of the circumcorneal blood vessels. This may occur acutely due to bacterial infection or Reiter's syndrome or be chronic as in syphilis, tuberculosis, sarcoidosis, sympathetic ophthalmitis, and ankylosing spondylitis. In diabetes mellitus, rubico iriditis may occur. |
| *Uveitis* | With uveitis that affects primarily the choroid, the eye is painless and the patient complains only of deteriorating vision. Uveitis occurs in sarcoidosis, ankylosing spondylitis, ulcerative colitis, Reiter's syndrome, rheumatoid arthritis, tuberculosis and syphilis. |

## Cornea

| | |
|---|---|
| *Keratitis* | Keratitis is painful and associated with a circumcorneal injection, which may be slight. |
| *Corneal ulceration* | It may progress to corneal ulceration which may be marginal, such as in staphylococcal infection, or central, related to foreign bodies, abrasion or dendritic ulcers. Congenital syphilis is associated with bilateral keratitis. |
| *Kerato-conjunctivitis sicca* | Abnormal dryness of the eyes, seen in Sjögren's syndrome, may also cause keratitis (kerato-conjunctivitis sicca). Schirmer's test can be used to confirm this. |
| *Arcus cornealis* | A white ring at the outer margin of the cornea probably represents continued exposure to high blood lipid levels. |
| *Kayser–Fleischer rings (rare)* | Kayser–Fleischer rings are seen in Wilson's disease (see Ch. 13). |

| | |
|---|---|
| *Calcification* | Bands or flecks of calcification may be found in association with chronic hypercalcaemia. |

## Pupils

| | |
|---|---|
| *Size/shape/ symmetry/reactivity* | The pupils should be inspected with a bright light and their size, shape, symmetry and reactivity to light noted. The light reflex is tested by shining a bright light from the side, avoiding the front which may provoke a convergence reaction. Both direct and consensual reactions should be tested in both eyes. Finally, accommodation should be checked, asking the patient to look at near and far objects. |
| *Argyll Robertson* | The Argyll Robertson pupil is small and irregular and reacts to accommodation but not to light. |
| *Holmes–Adie* | The Holmes–Adie pupil, on the other hand, is large and reacts sluggishly to light and accommodation. It may be associated with absent tendon reflexes, and is said to occur more commonly in women. |
| *Horner's syndrome* | In Horner's syndrome, the pupil is constricted and associated with partial ptosis, enophthalmos and ipsilateral anhydrosis. It is due to a lesion in the cervical sympathetic chain. |
| *Constriction* | Miosis (constricted pupils) is seen in iritis, opiate use, pontine lesions and with corneal or conjunctival irritation. |
| *Dilatation* | Bilateral dilatation of the pupils is frequently due to anxiety. Unilateral pupillary dilatation may be due to an amblyopic eye, third cranial nerve lesion, acute glaucoma, Holmes–Adie pupil, mydriatic drops and multiple sclerosis. |
| *Cataracts* | Cataracts, although best seen with the ophthalmoscope, are frequently visible using the torch, shining the beam of light tangentially. |
| **Ophthalmoscopy** | Although ophthalmoscopy is a technique of inspection, it is usually left to the end of the examination (see p. 23). |
| **Eye Movements** | Eye movements should be checked with the patient's head held steady with one hand, using the other as a moving target on which the patient fixes attention. Movement should be checked in vertical and horizontal planes. The |

corneal light reflections should be watched as their relative positions alter if one eye moves abnormally.

*Diplopia*　Ask specifically about diplopia and in what direction it is maximal. The eye responsible for the more peripheral image is the affected eye.

*Pain*　Pain associated with eye movement may suggest optic neuritis.

*Nystagmus*　Nystagmus should be looked for also during this procedure. For this reason, the target finger must be held at least 50 cm from the patient's eyes and the extremes of lateral gaze avoided. Nystagmus that is not maintained for 5 seconds is probably not significant (commenting on 'a few nystagmoid jerks' should be avoided in examinations). If nystagmus is identified, it should be described as pendular, rotary or jerking. If jerking, the direction of the rapid phase is used to describe the direction of nystagmus, and the direction of gaze at which it is maximal noted.

*Vertigo*　Associated symptoms such as vertigo should be recorded.

*Ataxic nystagmus*　Ataxic nystagmus (internuclear ophthalmoplegia) is characterised by nystagmus of the abducted eye and restricted adduction of the medial looking eye. It is relatively common in examinations and is nearly always due to multiple sclerosis.

*Conjugate deviation*　Failure of upward conjugate deviation can occur in disorders of the extra-pyramidal system (e.g. progressive supranuclear palsy and Parkinson's disease).

**Visual Fields**

*Confrontation*　The visual fields should be assessed by confrontation. The examiner should sit opposite the patient, approximately 1 metre away, and cover one of the patient's eyes. The patient should fix on the examiner's opposite eye. The peripheral visual fields are then assessed by moving a target into the field of vision from upper and lower, medial and lateral quadrants. The patient's visual field is checked against the examiner's. The moving target used is usually the examiner's index finger although use of red and white hat pins is more accurate.

| Menace reflex | In subjects who cannot cooperate with this test (e.g. drowsy or unconscious subjects), the menace reflex can be useful and is elicited by the examiner bringing his hand rapidly towards the patient's eye from his lateral field of vision and reflex blinking identified. Common visual field abnormalities are described in Table 3.1. |

**Table 3.1** Visual field abnormalities

| Field Loss | Site of Lesion |
| --- | --- |
| Total field loss from one eye | Retina or optic nerve |
| Bitemporal hemianopia | Optic chiasma |
| Non-congruous hemianopia | Optic tract |
| Upper homonymous quadrantanopia | Optic radiation (temporal) |
| Lower homonymous quadrantanopia | Optic radiation (parietal) |
| Homonymous hemianopia with macular sparing | Occipital cortex |
| Inattention hemianopia | Parietal lobe |
| Enlarged blind spot | Early papilloedema |
| Concentric constriction of field | Late papilloedema |
| Central scotoma (+ poor acuity) | Papillitis |

## Visual Acuity

| Print | The visual acuity can be assessed simply at the bedside by asking the patient to read newsprint of various sizes with each eye separately if a Snellen chart is unavailable. Patients should wear their glasses if these are usually worn |
| Finger counting and light recognition | for reading. If the acuity is very poor, the ability to count fingers or perceive light should be checked. |

| **AUSCULTATION** | Auscultation over the closed eye may reveal a bruit and should always be performed in patients with proptosis. In carotico-cavernous fistulae, pulsating exophthalmos is associated with a systolic bruit. |

| **PALPATION** | The intraocular pressure can be assessed approximately (with practice) by eliciting fluctuation over the downward looking eye. |

**OPHTHALMOSCOPY**

Ophthalmoscopy is usually carried out last. This examination is important and proficiency comes with practice. For a complete examination of the fundus, mydriatic drops must be used.

*Cornea*

Initially the cornea must be inspected with the ophthalmoscope held a few centimetres from the eye.

*Opacities*

Opacities in the cornea and anterior chamber, lens and vitreous will appear as black spots. Thereafter the instrument is brought close to the patient's eye and a suitable lens selected to bring the retina into focus.

*Cataract*

Cataracts are more readily apparent with the ophthalmoscope although they may be visible without. Causes include age, diabetes mellitus, Down's syndrome, post-infective (rubella, syphilis), drugs (e.g. steroids). Lens dislocation occurs in Marfan's syndrome, homocystinuria and trauma.

The following should be specifically inspected:

*Optic disc*
1. the optic disc, checking its size, shape, colour, margins and physiological cup

*Blood vessels*
2. retinal blood vessels, looking particularly at arterio-venous crossings and vessel calibre and tortuosity

*Retina*
3. background retina, looking for pigmentary abnormalities, exudates, haemorrhages and new vessels

*Periphery*
4. periphery, looking for pigmentary changes and retinal tears

*Macula*
5. the macular region, which is inspected last by asking the patient to look straight at the light. It is darker in colour and free of blood vessels. The central depression, the fovea, should be identified. Abnormalities in this region are especially important and affect visual acuity. Familiarity with typical hypertensive and diabetic retinopathies is essential for examinations. Common fundal changes are described in Table 3.2.

**Table 3.2** Fundal changes in common conditions

| Condition | Features | Causes |
|---|---|---|
| Papilloedema | Hyperaemia of disc<br>Obliteration of cup<br>Congestion of veins and loss of pulsation<br>Haemorrhages radiating from disc | Malignant hypertension<br>Raised IC pressure<br>Central retinal vein obstruction<br>$CO_2$ retention |
| Papillitis | Similar to papilloedema | Retrobulbar neuritis |
| Optic atrophy | Pale disc, blurred edge<br>Pale disc, sharp edge | Secondary to papilloedema<br>Retrobulbar neuritis<br>Optic nerve pressure<br>Diabetes mellitus<br>Retinal vein occlusion |
| Myelinated nerve fibres | Streaky irregular white patches adjacent to disc margin | Normal variant |
| Angioid streaks | Streaks across retina resembling blood vessels | Paget's disease<br>Pseudoxanthoma elasticum<br>Hyperphosphataemia<br>Acromegaly |
| Diabetes mellitus (Background) | Venous dilatation and tortuosity<br>Microaneurysms<br>Blot haemorrhages<br>Soft exudates (cotton-wool spots) | Both insulin dependent and non insulin dependent diabetes mellitus |
| (Proliferative) | New vessel formation<br>Vitreous haemorrhage<br>Retinal detachment<br>Retinitis proliferans | |
| Hypertension | Tortuous arteries<br>a-v nipping<br>Varying vessel calibre<br>Flame haemorrhages<br>Hard exudates<br>Papilloedema | Hypertension—<br>(Grades I &II)<br><br>(Grade III)<br><br>(Grade IV) |
| Anaemia | Pale background, engorged blood vessels, flame-shaped haemorrhages; woolly exudates | Severe anaemia of any cause especially pernicious anaemia, and leukaemia |
| Glaucoma | Increased cupping of the disc | In both open-angle and angle-closure forms |

# 4. CRANIAL NERVES

When examining cranial nerves it is often necessary to think of particular syndromes or conditions and to elicit additional or confirmatory signs affecting various cranial nerves or other parts of the body.

## I Olfactory

*Anosmia*

The sense of smell can be tested when appropriate with various scents (e.g. coffee, peppermint, vanilla), testing each nostril separately. Anosmia may be due to a frontal lobe tumour, meningioma, skull fracture, or Kallman's syndrome and may occur early in Alzheimer's disease.

## II, III, IV & VI

The testing of these cranial nerves is covered in Chapter 3.

## V Trigeminal

*Muscles of mastication*

Inspect the muscles of mastication (temporalis and masseter) and palpate the masseters when the patient's teeth are clenched.

*Pterygoid*

Ask the patient to open and close jaw against resistance. The jaw will move towards the side of a weakened pterygoid muscle. Bilateral weakness may occur in myasthenia gravis and some myopathies, e.g. dystrophia myotonica.

*Jaw jerk*

The jaw jerk is brisk in upper motor neurone lesions.

*Corneal reflex*

The corneal reflex is a useful test as it may be impaired in trigeminal nerve damage. It must, however, be tested carefully. The cornea should be lightly touched with a wisp of cotton wool, being careful to approach the eye laterally, out of the field of vision. Ask the patient if each side feels equally unpleasant (V nerve), and watch for asymmetry of eye closure in response (orbicularis oculi—VII nerve).

*Sensation*
Light touch and pinprick sensation should be tested comparing each side of the forehead, cheeks and jaws, thereby testing the three divisions of the trigeminal nerve.

## VII Facial

In addition to identifying the side affected, it must also be classified as upper or lower motor neurone in type.

*Facial muscles*
Voluntary contractions of the facial muscles should be examined and the two sides compared. Ask the patient to frown, raise eyebrows, wrinkle forehead, close eyes, puff out cheeks, show teeth (not 'smile' which is an emotional response) and whistle. Unilateral upper motor neurone lesions relatively spare the forehead, while lower motor neurone lesions involve the whole face.

*Bell's sign*
Bell's sign, an exaggerated upward movement of the eyeball on attempted eye closure, is seen in lower motor neurone lesions.

*Myasthenia (rare)*
Repeated testing of facial muscles may show progressive weakening in myasthenia gravis.

*Sensation*
Traditionally, taste sensation over the anterior two-thirds of the tongue is tested using sugar, salt, vinegar and quinine on each side of the tongue. The mouth should be rinsed between each test. However, touching the tongue with the terminals of a small transistor battery can be a good guide to loss of sensation.

*Glabellar tap*
The glabellar tap, repeated percussion over the root of the nose, shows attenuation of blinking in normal subjects, but not in parkinsonism. The presence of this feature is not diagnostic.

*Snout reflex*
The snout reflex, puckering or protrusion of the lips, is elicited by stroking the upper lip and is positive in frontal lobe disease or bilateral facial nerve upper motor neurone lesions.

*Hyperacusis*
Hyperacusis occurs in geniculate ganglion lesions due to paralysis of the stapedius muscle.

## VIII Auditory

*Hearing*
A rough assessment of hearing may be made by whispering in, or holding a ticking watch near to

each ear. The opposite external meatus should be occluded by a finger during testing.

*Rinne's test*  Rinne's test is performed using a high-pitched (256 Hz) tuning fork initially placed near the ear and then applied to the mastoid. Air conduction is louder than bone conduction in normal subjects and in nerve deafness; bone conduction is louder in conductive deafness.

*Weber's test*  Weber's test is performed by applying a tuning fork to the middle of the forehead. Normally the sound is heard in the midline. It is heard on the affected side in conduction or middle ear deafness and on the unaffected side in nerve or inner ear deafness.

*Auroscopy*  Auroscopy of external auditory meatus, looking for wax, signs of infection or a foreign body, should be carried out and then the tympanic membrane inspected for perforation, redness or deformity.

## VIII Vestibular

The vestibular part of the VIII nerve is usually tested only when indicated.

*Nystagmus*  Nystagmus should be looked for when testing eye movements. Positional nystagmus should be tested by lowering the patient's head off the bed below the horizontal and turning the head. The nystagmus produced is persistent in brain stem and cerebellar lesions but with time reduces with damage to the otolithic apparatus. (See also Ch. 19).

## IX Glossopharyngeal

*Gag reflex*  Touching the posterior wall of the pharynx with a tongue depressor evokes the gag reflex and tests the glossopharyngeal nerve.

*Palatal reflex*  The palatal reflex is more pleasant for the patient and is elicited by touching each side of the palate with an orange stick in turn. Taste to posterior third of tongue is difficult to test.

## X Vagus

*Palatal movement*  Palatal movement is assessed by asking the patient to say 'Ah'. The palate and uvula are pulled away from the weakened side.

| | |
|---|---|
| *Dysphagia* | Swallowing should be checked. Only drops of water from a syringe should be used if there is a question of dysphagia and the presence of a gag reflex sought. |
| *Dysphonia* | Dysphonia may be due to recurrent laryngeal nerve palsy and if present the vocal cords should be examined by indirect laryngoscopy using a laryngeal mirror. |

**XI Accessory**    The accessory nerve is tested by assessing the power of the trapezius and sternomastoid muscles against resistance. Turning the head away from the affected side is weakened in accessory nerve palsy. Bilateral weakness of the trapezius is seen in poliomyelitis and motor neurone disease whilst weakness of the sternomastoid occurs in muscular dystrophy, dystrophia myotonica and motor neurone disease. Spurious weakness with neck pain can occur in cervical spondylosis.

**XII Hypoglossal**    The tongue resting in the mouth should be inspected for fasciculation and wasting in lower motor neurone lesions. The tongue deviates towards the affected side on voluntary protrusion. In bilateral upper motor neurone lesions, tongue movement is sluggish. The protruded tongue should be moved from side to side; in pseudobulbar palsy due to cerebrovascular disease or motor neurone disease the speed of lateral movements may be diminished.

Rapid protrusion and retraction of the tongue (trombone tremor) occurs in Parkinsonism and in general paralysis of the insane. Continuous rotatory movements of the tongue may be drug induced (e.g. phenothiazines).

# 5. NECK

**INSPECTION**

The general appearance of the patient should be noted, particularly for evidence of thyrotoxicosis or myxoedema. Inspection of the neck should be carried out from the front, back and both sides, in good light, with adequate exposure of the neck and shoulders.

## Shape

*Short neck*

An abnormally short neck may indicate an underlying abnormality of the cervical spine such as the Klippel–Feil syndrome which may be associated with compression of the cervical cord.

*Webbing*

Webbing of the neck is a classical feature of Turner's syndrome and other signs should be sought.

*Kyphosis*

Kyphosis may be noted with advancing years.

## Swellings

*Goitre*
*Cysts*
*Salivary glands*
*Lymph nodes*
*Carotid pulse*




*Buffalo hump*

Swellings such as goitre, branchial and thyroglossal cysts, cystic hygroma, salivary gland enlargement and lymphadenopathy should be noted. A thyroglossal cyst rises on swallowing. Expansile carotid pulsation may be seen on the right side of the neck due to a kinked carotid artery, which is related to aortic unfolding and hypertension, or an aneurysm. The abnormality on inspection may be restricted to the back of the neck, e.g. the buffalo hump of Cushing's syndrome. The nature of all swellings should be confirmed, later, by palpation.

**Scars**

Scars of thyroid and parathyroid surgery should be looked for and their age estimated; if recent, latent tetany may be demonstrated as a positive

Chvostek's or Trousseau's sign. The irregular scars of scrofula may be present, and indicate past tuberculous involvement of the cervical lymph nodes.

**Skin**

*Vitiligo*

*Pseudoxanthoma elasticum (rare)*

*Spider naevi*

*Scleroderma*

The skin should be inspected for vitiligo (associated with autoimmune disease) and the 'plucked chicken' appearance of pseudoxanthoma elasticum (associated with arthropathy). Spider naevi may be prominent on the neck. A total of more than four should lead to a search for other signs of liver disease (see Ch. 8). Tightening of the skin of the neck may suggest systemic sclerosis.

**Jugular Venous Pulse**

The jugular venous pulse (JVP) which refers to the internal jugular vein should be looked for with the patient reclining at 45° with the neck relaxed. It is seen welling up between the heads of the sternomastoid. It is possible to use the external jugular vein if the pulsation rises and falls freely. It may or may not be pulsatile. It can be differentiated from the carotid pulse by the following characteristics: it is only rarely palpable, is biphasic, rises and falls relatively slowly and rises if pressure is applied over the vein at the base of the neck or over the abdomen (hepatojugular reflux). This latter is particularly conspicuous in tricuspid regurgitation and may be absent in hepatic vein occlusion (Budd–Chiari syndrome). The vertical height of the column of blood above the sternal angle should be measured. The JVP may not be easy to recognise when the venous pressure is grossly elevated (look for ear lobe pulsation) and may only become clearly visible when the patient is erect. A rough guide to the height of the JVP is to check the level at which the veins in the elevated arm collapse. The character of the venous pulsation should be assessed. Characteristic wave forms are shown in Figure 5.1.

*Kussmaul's sign*

Elevation of the JVP with inspiration is known as Kussmaul's sign and occurs when there is

i) Normal

ii) Large 'v' and slow 'x' descent –
    tricuspid regurgitation
    (confirm with pulsatile liver)

iii) Large 'a' - TS, PS, pulmonary
     hypertension (look for signs of RVH).
     Complete heart block (Cannon wave)

iv) Deep 'y' descent –
    constrictive pericarditis

v) Absent 'a' – atrial fibrillation

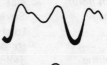

**Fig. 5.1** Characteristic jugular venous wave forms.

| | |
|---|---|
| *Constrictive pericarditis* | obstruction to venous filling of the heart as occurs in constrictive pericarditis. |
| *SVC obstruction* | A non-pulsatile JVP suggests superior vena caval obstruction; associated signs include oedema of the upper body, facial plethora and distension of superficial veins over the upper chest. The direction of flow in these veins should be ascertained and is downwards (towards the umbilicus) in superior vena caval obstruction. |

## Muscles

| | |
|---|---|
| *Accessory muscles of respiration* | Use of accessory muscles of respiration may be obvious in obstructive airways disease. |
| *Sternomastoid wasting* | Sternomastoid wasting is a hallmark of dystrophia myotonica. |
| *Torticollis* | Torticollis or wryneck may be obvious and if chronic may produce facial asymmetry. The patient should be asked to touch each shoulder in turn with both chin and ear to identify limitation of movement. |
| *Sternomastoid tumour* | In infancy a hard nodule within the sternomastoid muscle is referred to as a sternomastoid tumour. |

---

**PALPATION**    Palpation of the back and sides of the neck should be performed from in front of the patient.

## Thyroid Swellings

*Goitre*

Palpation of a goitre should be bimanual and is customarily done from behind the patient, with the patient's head in a neutral or even slightly flexed position. The texture of the gland (smooth or nodular, hard or soft) should be noted as well as its size. Confirmation of a swelling in the neck being thyroid or related to it, is made by asking the patient to swallow. (A glass of water should be provided if you ask the patient to swallow more than once.)

*Graves' disease*

Enlargement of the gland may be diffuse (Graves' disease, autoimmune thyroiditis and simple goitre), or nodular (toxic nodular, late simple goitre and carcinoma).

*Carcinoma*
*Viral thyroiditis*

Tenderness is characteristic of viral thyroiditis, but can be seen in autoimmune thyroiditis and carcinoma. Attachment of the gland to surrounding tissue suggests malignancy. Retrosternal extension of a goitre should be checked for by palpation in the suprasternal notch and by sternal percussion.

## Subcutaneous Emphysema

The characteristic crackling sensation of subcutaneous emphysema (gas within the tissues) may be felt on palpation and is associated with trauma, most frequently a fractured rib puncturing the lung, rupture of the oesophagus, or, rarely, gas gangrene.

## Salivary Glands

*Parotid*

Parotid gland enlargement is usually bilateral in acute inflammatory conditions, most commonly mumps. They may be enlarged in diabetes mellitus and debilitated alcoholic patients. Tuberculosis, sarcoidosis, Sjögren's syndrome, syphilis and lymphoma can cause unilateral or bilateral enlargement. Unilateral parotid swelling may be due to a 'mixed' parotid tumour which can grow to considerable size. Intermittent swelling may be caused by duct calculi. The parotid duct opening, opposite the second upper molars, must be examined. Reddening around the opening is seen in mumps and pus may be expressed in suppurative parotitis. Mikulicz's syndrome is characterised by enlargement of salivary and lacrimal glands and xerostomia. Parotid enlargement may be associated with a LMN VII nerve palsy, e.g. in 'mixed' parotid tumour, tuberculosis, syphilis, lymphoma, and leukaemia. Uveo-parotid syndrome is parotid enlargement, iridocyclitis with or without choroiditis.

*Submandibular*
Enlargement of the submandibular glands is rare, but should be checked for as swelling beneath and anterior to the angle of the jaw. Swelling that is intermittent and related to meals is due to Wharton's submandibular duct obstruction.

**Lymphadenopathy**
The neck should be palpated systematically. From the front palpate the back and sides of the neck. Thereafter, sit the patient forward and continue palpation from behind: begin superiorly and examine the submandibular and tonsilar lymph nodes, continue over the anterior and posterior triangles of the neck, and conclude by palpating above the clavicles and deep to the sternoclavicular insertions of the sternomastoids. It is important to include all salivary glands and lymph nodes (Fig. 5.2). Cervical nodes are sometimes more easily palpable when the patient performs a Valsalva manoeuvre. Lymphadenopathy may be localised or generalised and generally reflects either infection or malignancy.

*Localised*
*Generalised*

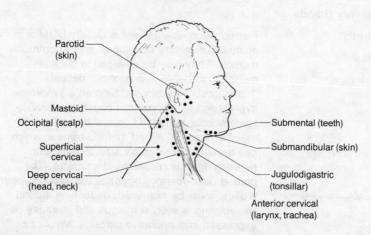

Parotid (skin)

Mastoid

Occipital (scalp)

Superficial cervical

Deep cervical (head, neck)

Submental (teeth)

Submandibular (skin)

Jugulodigastric (tonsillar)

Anterior cervical (larynx, trachea)

**Fig. 5.2** Lymph nodes of the neck (and areas of drainage).

Primary
Secondary
Malignancy

Malignancy may be primary (lymphoma or leukaemia) or secondary and attention should be paid to the tongue, throat, nose and paranasal sinuses as well as more readily apparent areas when deciding the origin of the lymphadenopathy. Generalised lymphadenopathy may be a presenting feature of HIV infection (see Ch. 22).

Troisier's sign

Enlargement of the left supraclavicular lymph nodes (Virchow's node) may indicate a carcinoma of the stomach is present (Troisier's sign).

A 10-point checklist of any swelling should be made (see Table 5.1) and will assist in the interpretation of the problem. Swellings in neighbouring tissues and regional lymph nodes should be sought and usually indicate spread of infection or tumour.

**Table 5.1**    10-point checklist for swellings

1. Size
2. Shape
3. Surface texture
4. Colour
5. Consistency
6. Margins
7. Mobility
8. Position
9. Tenderness
10. Temperature

**Trachea**

Deviation
Length
Tug

} See Chapter 7.

Tracheal 'tug' may be felt in airways obstruction or with a syphilitic aortic aneurysm.

**Carotid Pulse**

The carotid pulses should be palpated with the thumb (one side at a time only) and the rate, rhythm, volume and character noted (see Ch. 6).

Corrigan's sign

An easily visible carotid pulsation in aortic regurgitation is known as Corrigan's sign. A visible carotid pulse may also be seen in older patients and may be due to arteriosclerosis or aneurysmal dilation. In the young, an obvious arterial pulse in the suprasternal notch should suggest coarctation of the aorta.

## PERCUSSION

| | |
|---|---|
| *Retrosternal goitre* | A retrosternal goitre may be identified by percussion, though percussion of the neck is not routinely carried out. |

## AUSCULTATION

### Bruit

| | |
|---|---|
| *Goitre* | A bruit may be heard over a goitre and usually indicates thyrotoxicosis as opposed to a non-toxic goitre. Do not confuse with a venous hum. |
| *Carotid* | Vascular bruits from carotid or subclavian stenosis may be heard in the neck as may |
| *Radiated cardiac murmurs* | radiated cardiac murmurs, particularly aortic stenosis. Carotid bruits should lead to a search for signs of a stroke. |
| *Venous hum* | A venous hum may be heard above either clavicle in a sitting or reclining patient but is not heard in supine subjects. It is commoner in children. Its intensity varies with head movement and can be abolished by pressure on the neck above the stethoscope. |
| *Subcutaneous emphysema* | When subcutaneous emphysema is suspected, auscultation over the suspected area may enable crackling to be heard when crepitus is difficult to feel. |

# 6. CARDIOVASCULAR SYSTEM

After examining the cardiovascular system you should be able to:
1. describe the pathological abnormality (ies) present
2. describe the functional effect these have had
3. describe additional confirmatory signs.

| | |
|---|---|
| **GENERAL INSPECTION** | It is helpful to note general changes first. |
| *Pallor* | Pallor may suggest shock due to myocardial infarction or pulmonary embolus, or anaemia which can itself cause a tachycardia and worsening of cardiac failure, or can be due to infective endocarditis. |
| *Dresden doll face* | A pale appearance likened to a Dresden china doll's is sometimes seen with aortic stenosis. |
| *Anxiety* | An anxious appearance may suggest underlying thyrotoxicosis or phaeochromocytoma, while an anxiety state may cause a tachycardia and a raised jugular venous pressure. |
| *Sweating* | A 'cold' sweat is a common accompaniment of myocardial infarction. |
| *Peripheral cyanosis* | Cyanosis, which may be peripheral or central, (see Ch. 12) should be noted; peripheral cyanosis with cold extremities suggests a low output state while central cyanosis may be due to right-to-left cardiac shunts or cor pulmonale. |
| *Breathlessness* | Acute breathlessness may accompany a myocardial infarction, left ventricular failure or pulmonary embolus, while chronic breathlessness may suggest cor pulmonale, which is commonly secondary to chronic obstructive airways disease. |

| | |
|---|---|
| *Orthopnoea* | Orthopnoea, breathlessness induced by lying flat, is a sign of incipient left ventricular failure. |

**Face**

| | |
|---|---|
| *Mitral facies* | Mitral facies, a bluish discoloration of the cheeks is seen in mitral stenosis, but is not specific to the disease. A 'peaches and cream' complexion with fullness of the face should alert one to |
| *Myxoedema* | myxoedema. |
| *Polycythaemia* | High colour of the face, sometimes with suffusion of the conjunctivae, is seen in polycythaemia but is more often related to outdoor exposure. |
| *Down's syndrome* | The typical facial appearance of Down's syndrome should alert the examiner to the possibility of an atrial septal defect (ostium primum). |
| *Head nodding* | Nodding of the head in time with the arterial pulse is sometimes seen in aortic regurgitation (De Mussett's sign) and should be differentiated from titubation or Parkinsonism. |
| *Argyll Robertson pupils* | Argyll Robertson pupils are seen in tertiary syphilis and may be associated with aortic regurgitation. |
| *Arcus cornealis* | Arcus cornealis is associated with hyperlipidaemia. |
| *Lens dislocation* | Lens dislocation may be seen in Marfan's |
| *High arched palate* | syndrome as may a high arched palate (also seen in supravalvular aortic stenosis). |

**Hands and Legs**   Careful examination of the hands may also provide helpful clues.

| | |
|---|---|
| *Finger clubbing* | Finger clubbing is seen in cyanotic congenital heart disease and infective endocarditis or may suggest underlying chest disease (see Ch. 7). |
| *Palmar creases* | Pallid palmar creases suggest anaemia and may help differentiate from the general pallor of shock. |
| *Splinters* | Splinter haemorrhages are seen in infective |
| *Osler's nodes (rare)* | endocarditis as are Osler's nodes (tender palpable |
| *Janeway lesions (rare)* | nodules in the pulps of the fingertips), Janeway lesions (palpable purpuric spots on the palm) and necrotic lesions due to emboli. |
| *Rheumatoid deformity* | Rheumatoid deformity of the hands and rheumatoid nodules around the elbows should alert the examiner to cardiac involvement such as pericarditis and cardiomyopathy. |
| *Scleroderma* | Atrophy of the fingertips with or without infarction should suggest systemic sclerosis |

which may also affect the heart. Soft tissue calcification may be present.

*Capillary pulsations*   Exaggerated nail bed capillary pulsations elucidated by slight pressure distally over the nails is seen in aortic regurgitation (Quincke's pulse).

*Arachnodactyly*   Arachnodactyly is seen in Marfan's syndrome which is associated with aortic regurgitation, mitral regurgitation, aortic dissection and cardiac conduction abnormalities.

*Xanthomas*   Tendon xanthomas occur in familial hyper-chole sterolaemia (Type IIa), as well as xanthelasma and arcus cornealis. Palmar xanthomas occur in Type III and eruptive xanthomas in Type V.

*Oedema*   Peripheral oedema over both feet and ankles is typical of congestive cardiac failure, but also occurs in association with hypoalbuminaemia and inferior vena caval obstruction. In congestive cardiac failure and hypoproteinaemia, fluid tends to collect in the most dependent part of the body. Sacral oedema therefore must be looked for in bed-bound patients.

*Deep venous thrombosis*   Swelling also occurs with a deep venous thrombosis with associated signs of erythema, tenderness, dilated superficial veins and increased skin temperature.

*Baker's cyst*   Baker's cyst should be considered in the differential diagnosis.

**Neck**   Inspection of the neck, and the jugular venous pressure in particular, is conventionally performed after palpating the peripheral pulses (See Ch. 5)

**Chest**

*Café au lait*   Café au lait patches can occur in infective endocarditis and neurofibromatosis.

*Pectus excavatum*   Pectus excavatum or funnel chest deformity is relatively common and can cause displacement of the heart.

*Pectus carinatum*   Pectus carinatum or pigeon chest and prominent Harrison's sulci are seen in rickets.

*Median sternotomy*   A median sternotomy scar may indicate surgery for valvular or ischaemic heart disease.

*Left parasternal impulse*   A left parasternal impulse is sometimes visible in right ventricular hypertrophy.

| | |
|---|---|
| *Apex beat* | The apex beat can be seen sometimes in thin individuals and is more prominent with hyperdynamic states. |
| *Kyphoscoliosis* | Kyphoscoliotic deformities of the spine can cause displacement of the heart and cardiac failure, while the rigid kyphotic back of ankylosing spondylitis should alert to the possibility of aortic regurgitation. |
| *Straight back* | The rigid straight spine of the straight back syndrome is associated with a parasternal systolic murmur. |

## Abdomen

| | |
|---|---|
| *Ascites* | Abdominal distension due to ascites may occur in severe congestive cardiac failure and constrictive pericarditis. |
| *Aortic pulsation* | Although pulsation in the upper abdomen is common in healthy, thin subjects, it may be obvious in patients with an aortic aneurysm. |

## PALPATION

| | |
|---|---|
| *Skin temperature* | The skin temperature, especially of the hands and feet, should be noted and an assessment made of the peripheral circulation. |
| *Capillary filling* | The speed of return of capillary filling following blanching produced by applying pressure over the skin of the fingers, toes and earlobes is frequently used to assess the adequacy of the |
| *Peripheral pulses* | peripheral circulation, as well as checking for the presence of peripheral pulses. |

| | |
|---|---|
| **Pulse** **Rate** | Normally the radial pulse is checked first and the rate determined. |
| *Sinus bradycardia* | Physiological variation in the heart rate is 60–100 beats per minute. A slower heart rate may be due to a sinus bradycardia (40–60) which occurs in athletes, post-myocardial infarction, hypothyroidism, hypothermia, raised intra-cranial pressure and those taking beta blockers. |
| *Complete heart block* | In complete heart block the rate is usually slower (30–45) and associated with Cannon waves seen in the jugular venous pulse. It may complicate mycocardial infarction and cardiomyopathy or be drug-induced or idiopathic. |

| | |
|---|---|
| *Sinus tachycardia* | A rapid heart rate may be due to sinus tachycardia (> 100) which may be seen in anxiety, cardiac failure, fever, anaemia, thyrotoxicosis, and children, or to a |
| *Supraventricular tachycardia* | supraventricular tachycardia (120–200) which is frequently paroxysmal and idiopathic but may be due to thyrotoxicosis, ischaemic heart disease, excess tobacco and caffeine or pre-excitation syndromes (Wolff–Parkinson–White and Lown–Ganong–Levine). Carotid sinus massage may restore sinus rhythm in supraventricular |
| *Atrial flutter* | tachycardia. Atrial flutter with 2:1 block (150) may slow in a stepwise fashion during carotid pressure (150→100→75) and is associated with ischaemic heart disease, thyrotoxicosis and digoxin toxicity. |

**Rhythm**

The rhythm should also be determined from the radial pulse — the rhythms described above are all regular.

*Irregular*
*Sinus arrhythmia*
*Ventricular ectopics*

Irregularities may be due to sinus arrhythmia (variation with respiration — common in young adults) or multiple ventricular ectopic beats (seen in ischaemia, thyrotoxicosis and cardiomyopathy), in which case the rhythm may become regular after exercise.

*Coupled beats*
*Dropped beats*

Coupled beats (bigemini) are characteristic of digoxin toxicity whilst true 'dropped beats' occur in second degree heart block.

*Atrial flutter*
*Atrial fibrillation*

Atrial flutter with variable block may be intermittently irregular while atrial fibrillation, which complicates hypertension, ischaemia, rheumatic heart disease and thyrotoxicosis, or, more rarely, pulmonary embolus, alcoholic cardiomyopathy and pericarditis, is 'irregularly irregular'. Atrial fibrillation does not become regular with exercise. A pulse deficit between radial and apical rates may be noted.

*Ventricular tachycardia*
*Ventricular fibrillation*

The pulse in ventricular tachycardia (120–200) is irregular and frequently feeble. No pulse is felt in either ventricular fibrillation or asystole.

*Radial pulse*

An absent radial pulse may be a congenital abnormality or due to arterial embolism or a Blalock shunt.

**Character and Volume**

The character and volume of the pulse is best assessed at the carotid artery, using the thumb.

| | |
|---|---|
| *Plateau pulse* | A low volume pulse which slowly rises and falls (plateau pulse) is seen in aortic stenosis. |
| *Low volume* | Other causes of a low volume pulse include mitral stenosis, pulmonary hypertension and shock. |
| *High volume*<br>*Collapsing pulse* | A high volume pulse which rapidly rises then falls away abruptly (collapsing pulse) is seen particularly in aortic regurgitation but found also with high cardiac output states such as patent ductus arteriosus, pregnancy, a-v malformations, severe anaemia, hypercapnia, hepatic cirrhosis, fever, thyrotoxicosis, rarely in Paget's disease, and also in complete heart block. It can be demonstrated at the wrist by placing the palm of the right hand over the radial artery and then elevating the patient's arm, keeping his elbow straight with your left hand. The pulse volume increases on elevation in patients with a collapsing pulse. |
| *Jerky* | A jerky upstroke is characteristic of hypertrophic obstructive cardiomyopathy. This condition can also produce the double beat (bisferiens) which is found more typically in combined aortic stenosis and regurgitation. |
| *Bisferiens* | |
| *Dicrotic* | An apparent second impulse with each beat (dicrotic) is felt in fever and hyperdynamic states. |
| *Alternans* | Alternating high and low volume beats (alternans) sometimes accompany left ventricular failure and may be confirmed using the sphygmomanometer. The volume of the pulse normally decreases slightly on inspiration but this is exaggerated (so-called paradoxus) in cardiac tamponade, constrictive pericarditis and severe airways obstruction. |
| *Paradoxus* | |
| *Inequality* | Inequality between the radial pulses may be seen in Takayasu's disease and aortic aneurysm, whilst an absent radial pulse may suggest an embolus. |
| *Absent radial* | |
| *Radiofemoral delay* | Delay in pulse transmission to the femoral arteries is found in coarctation of the aorta. |
| **Blood pressure** | The blood pressure, which must always be recorded in the cardiovascular examination, often confirms findings suspected from the character of the pulse. This recording may be left to the end of the examination. |

**Neck**

| | |
|---|---|
| *Jugular venous*<br>*pressure* | The jugular venous pulse should then be inspected (see Ch.5). |

## Precordium

| | |
|---|---|
| *Apex beat* | The apex beat, the furthest downward and outward point at which the cardiac impulse is palpable, should be located. It is normally in the fifth intercostal space at the midclavicular line. Count down from the sternal angle which lies beside the second rib. The patient should be lying straight when the apex beat is examined. |
| *Thrusting* | A thrusting, heaving or sustained apex beat is found with left ventricular hypertrophy. |
| *Tapping* | A tapping apex beat, due to a palpable first heart sound, may be found in mitral stenosis. |
| *Double impulse* | A dyskinetic or aneurysmal segment of the left ventricle may lead to a double or diffuse impulse. A double impulse may also occur in hypertrophic obstructive cardiomyopathy. |
| *Absent impulse* *Dextrocardia* | An absent apex beat may be due to pericardial effusion, obesity or emphysema; in dextrocardia the apex beat is found on the right side. |
| *Pericardial knock* | A pericardial 'knock' may occur in constrictive pericarditis. |
| *Parasternal heave* | A right ventricular heave should be sought in the left parasternal area and occurs in right ventricular hypertrophy. There may be a double kick when the right atrium is enlarged in mitral regurgitation. A palpable second heart sound occurs in pulmonary hypertension, whilst a pulsatile aortic arch aneurysm may be felt in the second right intercostal space. |
| *Apical thrills* | Apical thrills (palpable bruit) are systolic in mitral regurgitation and papillary muscle rupture and diastolic in mitral stenosis. |
| *Parasternal thrill* | A left parasternal thrill is associated with a ventricular septal defect. |
| *Basal thrills* | Thrills at the base of the heart again may be systolic in aortic or pulmonary stenosis or diastolic in aortic and pulmonary regurgitation. It is best to interpret thrills in combination with auscultatory findings. |

## Abdomen

| | |
|---|---|
| *Hepatomegaly* | Hepatomegaly should be sought and has a smooth, rounded edge in congestive cardiac failure and may be pulsatile with tricuspid regurgitation. |

## PERCUSSION

*Cardiac dullness*  The area of cardiac dullness is variable and of limited value. However, increased right parasternal dullness may be detected in pericardial effusion and left atrial enlargement, whilst the absence of cardiac dullness occurs in obesity and emphysema.

*Pleural effusions*  Pleural effusions, detected by percussion over the base of the chest, may occur, for example, in cardiac failure (see Ch. 7).

## AUSCULTATION

Auscultation of the heart (Fig. 6.1) should begin with the diaphragm of the stethoscope, listening in turn (1→8) at the apex, the axilla, the lower left parasternal area, the lower right parasternal area, the upper right parasternal area, the carotid arteries, the upper and mid left parasternal area (with the patient sitting forward in expiration) and finally with the bell at or just medial to the apex (with the patient turned on the left side and after exercise if necessary). Using this systematic approach, most sounds and murmurs will be identified.

### Heart Sounds

*First heart sound*  The first heart sound is due mainly to mitral
*Loud*  valve closure. It is loud in mitral stenosis and a
*Soft*  hyperdynamic circulation, and soft in mitral regurgitation, calcified mitral stenosis,

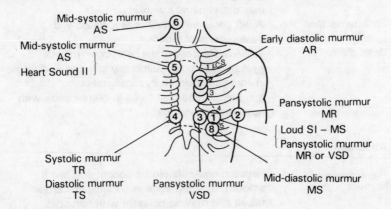

Mid-systolic murmur AS — ⑥

Mid-systolic murmur AS ⎫
Heart Sound II ⎭ ⑤

Early diastolic murmur AR

1 ICS

⑦
3

⑦

④ ③ ① ②
⑧ 5

Pansystolic murmur MR

{ Loud SI – MS
Pansystolic murmur MR or VSD

Systolic murmur TR
Diastolic murmur TS

Pansystolic murmur VSD

Mid-diastolic murmur MS

**Fig. 6.1**  Auscultation of the heart.

hypotension and severe heart failure. It varies in intensity in complete heart block and ventricular tachycardia.

*Split S1*                 The normal splitting of the first heart sound is more pronounced in right bundle branch block.

*Second heart sound*       The second heart sound is due to aortic and pulmonary valve closure and normally the aortic component occurs first in adults and is louder.

*Split S2*                 Splitting of the second sound diminishes in expiration, whilst wide splitting occurs in pulmonary stenosis and left bundle branch block.

*Fixed split*              Fixed splitting (no change with respiration) occurs with atrial septal defect and right bundle branch block.

*Reversed split*           Paradoxical or reversed splitting (pulmonary before aortic component and decreasing on inspiration) may occur in left bundle branch block, severe aortic stenosis, left ventricular failure and patent ductus arteriosus.

*Single S2*                A single second sound may be heard in calcified aortic stenosis, pulmonary stenosis and common truncus arteriosus as well as appearing single in some normal elderly patients.

*Third heart sound*        The third heart sound is due to ventricular filling at the time of a-v valve opening and is normal in young people towards the cardiac apex. It also occurs where there is rapid ventricular filling — mitral regurgitation, ventricular septal defect, congestive cardiac failure and constrictive pericarditis.

*Fourth heart sound*       The fourth heart sound is due to ventricular filling as a result of atrial contraction and is heard in cardiac failure, myocardial infarction, hypertension and hypertrophic obstructive cardiomyopathy.

*Gallop rhythm*            A gallop rhythm, a tachycardia with added third or fourth sound (or both — summation gallop) may be heard in heart failure.

*Opening snap*             Other added sounds include the opening snap
*Ejection click*           heard in mitral stenosis and an ejection click heard sometimes in aortic stenosis, hypertension, and mitral valve prolapse.

**Murmurs**                Cardiac murmurs are conventionally divided into systolic and diastolic and the loudness graded from 1 to 6:

1. just audible (in quiet surroundings)
2. quiet
3. moderately loud
4. loud with palpable thrill
5. very loud with pronounced thrill
6. audible without the aid of stethoscope.

As murmurs are sometimes graded from only 1 to 4 it is preferable always to indicate the scale used (e.g. 2/4 or 3/6). The characteristics of the commoner murmurs are listed in Table 6.1.

## Systolic
### Mid-systolic

*Innocent*

Innocent mid-systolic murmurs at the left sternal edge may be heard in hyperdynamic states, pregnancy and chest deformities.

*Aortic stenosis*

A mid-systolic murmur at the right upper sternal edge which radiates to the neck (and may radiate to the apex) is heard in aortic stenosis.

*Aortic sclerosis*

A similar murmur, sometimes with a mewing 'seagull's cry' quality, is heard in aortic sclerosis.

*Mitral valve prolapse*
*HOCM*
*Pulmonary stenosis*
*Atrial septal defect*

The mid-to-late systolic murmurs due to mitral valve prolapse or hypertrophic obstructive cardiomyopathy occur at the left sternal edge as do those of pulmonary stenosis and atrial septal defect.

### Pansystolic

*Mitral regurgitation*

*Ventricular septal defect*

*Ruptured chordae*

Pansystolic murmurs at the apex due to mitral regurgitation radiate to the axilla whilst those due to a ventricular septal defect radiate to the left sternal edge.
Systolic murmurs associated with rupture of chordae tendinae may radiate to the right upper chest.

*Tricuspid regurgitation*

Tricuspid regurgitation murmurs occur at the right lower sternal edge especially on inspiration and are associated with hepatic pulsation and giant jugular venous 'v' waves.

### Diastolic
### Early diastolic

*Aortic regurgitation*

The early diastolic murmur of aortic regurgitation

**Table 6.1.** Findings in common cardiac lesions

| Lesion | Murmur | Associated signs |
|---|---|---|
| Aortic stenosis | Mid-systolic at upper right sternal border (to neck/apex) | Thrill<br>Click<br>Faint aortic or single or reversed second sound<br>Thrusting apex<br>Plateau pulse<br>BP — low systolic, small pulse pressure<br>Pale complexion |
| Pulmonary stenosis | Mid-systolic at upper left sternal border | Cyanosis<br>RV heave<br>Split second sound (soft $P_2$)<br>JVP — large 'a' wave, small volume pulse |
| Aortic regurgitation | Blowing early diastolic at left sternal border | Thrusting displaced apex<br>Head nodding<br>Carotid pulsation<br>Collapsing pulse<br>BP — wide pulse pressure<br>Femoral bruit |
| Mitral stenosis | Rumbling mid-diastolic murmur at apex (plus pre-systolic except AF) | Palpable loud first sound<br>Opening snap<br>Mitral facies<br>Peripheral cyanosis<br>Small volume pulse, often AF |
| Mitral regurgitation | Pansystolic at apex (to axilla) | Thrusting displaced apex<br>Thrill<br>Third heart sound |
| VSD | Rough pansystolic at apex (to sternum) | No cyanosis (unless R→L shunt)<br>Thrill<br>Thrusting displaced apex |
| ASD | Pulmonary systolic | Fixed split second sound<br>RV heave |
| PDA | Continuous machinery murmur at upper left of sternum (to back) | Thrusting apex<br>BP — wide pulse pressure |
| Coarctation of aorta | Loud rough systolic at left lung apex, back and front | Scapular and internal mammary collaterals — bruits<br>Radiofemoral delay<br>Hypertension in arms |

*Pulmonary regurgitation*

may be heard at any position down the left sternal edge and is accentuated by expiration, while pulmonary regurgitation is accentuated by inspiration. An early diastolic murmur in the pulmonary area may be heard in pulmonary

| | |
|---|---|
| *Graham Steel (rare)* | hypertension due to mitral stenosis (Graham Steel). |

## Mid-diastolic

| | |
|---|---|
| *Mitral stenosis* | The mid-diastolic murmur of mitral stenosis is low-pitched and rumbling and heard at or just medial to the apex and may be accentuated by turning the patient on to the left side and by exercise (e.g. touching toes in bed). |
| *Pre-systolic accentuation* | A pre-systolic component to the murmur of mitral stenosis may be heard in sinus rhythm. An apical diastolic murmur is sometimes heard with |
| *Austin Flint (rare)* | aortic incompetence (Austin Flint). |
| *Tricuspid stenosis* | Tricuspid stenosis is rare and best heard at the right lower sternal edge. |
| *Carey Coombs* | A short diastolic murmur is heard with acute rheumatic mitral valvulitis (Carey Coombs). |

## Continuous

Continuous murmurs may be heard in coarctation of the aorta, arterio-venous shunts, patent ductus arteriosus and ruptured sinus of Valsalva. A venous hum simulates a continuous murmur and may be abolished by light pressure on the side of the neck.

**Posture**

It should be remembered that change in posture can influence murmurs. For example, rising from the sitting position decreases venous return and therefore reduces the murmur of pulmonary and aortic stenosis whilst increasing the murmur associated with mitral valve prolapse and hypertrophic obstructive cardiomyopathy. Squatting increases cardiac afterload and increases aortic, pulmonary and mitral regurgitation.

## Pericardial Rub

A creaky, 'leathery' sound may be heard in pericarditis, which may vary with respiration and posture. It may be systolic, diastolic or both. A pleuropericardial rub varies throughout the respiratory cycle.

## Other Bruits

Carotid bruits should be sought and differentiated from cardiac murmurs. Femoral bruits are usually due to atherosclerosis, but in aortic regurgitation a to-and-fro bruit may be produced by partially occluding the artery proximally (Duroziez's sign).

**Lungs**     Auscultation of the lung fields is essential, paying particular attention to the presence of crepitations and signs of chronic lung disease (see Ch. 7).

**Blood pressure**     The blood pressure should be recorded in both the erect and supine position with a sphygmomanometer cuff of adequate size around the arm at the level of the heart (see also Ch. 17). Korotkoff phase V is usually accepted as the diastolic pressure.

**Fundi**     The fundi should be examined for changes particularly in hypertension and infective endocarditis (Roth spots) (see Ch. 3).

# 7. RESPIRATORY SYSTEM

After examining the respiratory system you should be able to:
1. detect evidence of long-standing chest disease
2. detect abnormalities associated with an acute problem
3. describe the sequelae of your findings.

## INSPECTION

### Hands

It is conventional to start the examination of the respiratory system with the hands.

*Finger clubbing*

Finger clubbing (see Ch. 1) is an important clinical sign and occurs in association with certain pulmonary disorders, e.g. bronchiectasis, bronchial carcinoma, mesothelioma, asbestosis, empyema and fibrosing alveolitis.

*Asterixis*

A flapping tremor (asterixis) occurs in hypercapnia (see Ch. 1). Other signs of $CO_2$ retention are dilated veins, a bounding pulse, papilloedema, confusion and sweating.

*Bounding pulse*

*Peripheral cyanosis*

Peripheral cyanosis should be noted if present (see Ch. 12).

### Face

*Central cyanosis*
*Buccal mucosa*

Central cyanosis (see Ch. 12) is detected by inspecting the buccal mucosa and differentiates 'blue bloaters' from 'pink puffers' in chronic obstructive airways disease.

*Moon face*

A 'moon face' may be present and related to steroid therapy in obstructive airways disease.

### Eyes

*Horner's syndrome*

Horner's syndrome (see Ch. 3) in a patient with chest disease is an important finding and usually indicates involvement of the cervical sympathetic nerves by an apical bronchial carcinoma (Pancoast's syndrome).

## Chest and Neck

*Accessory muscles of respiration*

Use of the accessory muscles of respiration usually indicates respiratory difficulty. The patient frequently sits upright with arms extended supporting and fixing the chest thereby enabling these accessory muscles to help with respiration. A wheeze or stridor may be present.

## Chest Shape

*Straight back*

A straight or rigid back with decreased expansion is seen in ankylosing spondylosis.

*Scoliosis*

Scoliosis may be associated with rib or chest wall flattening and, if secondary to pulmonary disease, indicates a chronic disorder.

*Kyphosis*

Kyphosis may be severe enough (e.g. Pott's disease of spine) to impair respiration.

*Barrel chest*

Barrel deformity is an increase in anteroposterior diameter with thoracic kyphosis, ribs and clavicles more horizontal than usual, filling of supraclavicular fossa, and a subcostal angle greater than 90°, and is often associated with emphysema.

*Pectus carinatum*

Pectus carinatum or pigeon chest is an increased prominence of upper sternum often due to rickets (look for Harrison's sulcus) or chronic chest infection.

*Pectus excavatum*

Pectus excavatum or funnel chest is a depression of lower sternum, is usually congenital and perhaps due to a short central diaphragmatic tendon.

*Rickety rosary*
*Harrison's sulci*

Prominent costochondral epiphyses seen in rickets (rickety rosary), may be associated with Harrison's sulci, a deformity associated with indrawing of the ribs below the nipple due to traction of diaphragm. This latter deformity may be seen in childhood asthma as well as rickets.

*Intercostal indrawing*

Intercostal indrawing indicates increased negative intrathoracic pressure, usually associated with obstructive airways disease.

*Expansion*

Chest expansion is best inspected by observing the supine patient from the foot of the bed. Symmetry of expansion of both sides of chest should be checked.

| | |
|---|---|
| *Respiratory rate and pattern* | The normal respiratory rate is approximately 14/min; an increased rate (tachypnoea) is seen in anxiety states, painful and restrictive chest diseases (where it is often shallow), pneumonia, pulmonary embolism and left ventricular failure. Rapid and deep respiration is seen in states of metabolic acidosis such as diabetic ketoacidosis. Cheyne–Stokes respiration, cycles of increasing and decreasing depths of respiration, is seen in patients with cerebral or respiratory depression associated with cerebrovascular disease, uraemia, and cardiac failure. |
| **Sputum Pot** | The sputum pot should be inspected. |

## PALPATION

| | |
|---|---|
| *Mediastinal displacement* | Mediastinal displacement is checked by assessing the position of the trachea and apex beat. |
| *Tracheal deviation* | The tracheal position is the more important sign and should be checked in all patients. The neck should be slightly flexed and not rotated. Methods of assessing centrality include:<br>1. Insert the index and middle fingers into the suprasternal notch and feel for tracheal displacement *or*<br>2. Place the middle finger into the centre of the suprasternal notch with the second and fourth fingers on either side of the suprasternal notch feeling for the centre of the trachea *or*<br>3. Grip the trachea with the thumb and index finger and determine position. |
| *Apex beat* | The position of the apex beat should be noted, but it should be remembered that its position is influenced by heart size and displacement is only infrequently due to mediastinal displacement. The mediastinum is displaced to the left in collapse or fibrosis of left lower lobe, right pleural effusion or right pneumothorax and displaced to the right by left pneumothorax or pleural effusion, or fibrosis or collapse of the right lower lobe. |
| *Crico-sternal distance* | The distance between the cricoid cartilage and the sternal notch should be determined and is |

| | reduced in emphysema and during an asthmatic attack. |
|---|---|
| *Lymphadenopathy (Supraclavicular & Axillary)* | Supraclavicular (see Ch. 5) and axillary lymphadenopathy should be noted. |
| *Breasts* | The breasts should be inspected for symmetry and nipple indrawing or discharge and skin changes. Examine with the patient's hands by her side, on her hips and held behind her head. Palpate with the palmar aspect of the fingers in a rotary fashion exerting initially gentle and later firmer pressure against chest wall. Examine each quadrant in turn. |
| *Gynaecomastia* | Gynaecomastia is the presence of increased breast tissue in men. It should be differentiated from obesity by the granular texture of periareolar tissue. It may occur in liver disease, at puberty, in testicular teratomata and neoplasms such as carcinoma and lymphoma, in endocrine disorders such as hyperthyroidism, acromegaly and Addison's disease, Klinefelter's syndrome, renal failure and with drugs such as oestrogen, spironolactone, digoxin, methyldopa and cimetidine. |
| *Chest expansion* | Chest expansion should be measured as follows: the thumbs should be placed as vertical as is possible on either side of the midline with the fingers gripping firmly the patient's lateral chest wall; assess expansion anteriorly and posteriorly in upper and lower zones. Normal expansion should be at least 5 cm. Diminished expansion is seen with consolidation, atelectasis, lung abscess, fibrosis, pneumothorax and large pleural effusions. |
| *Tactile vocal fremitus* | Tactile vocal fremitus should be assessed with one hand on both sides of chest using the ulnar aspect of the cupped hand (or the palm) whilst the patient repeats the words '111' or '99'. Tactile vocal fremitus gives the same information as vocal resonance: increased in consolidation and reduced with pleural effusions and collapse. |

| **PERCUSSION** | Percussion of the chest should cover the upper, middle and lower segments — anteriorly, posteriorly and laterally. Two 'taps' are sufficient; the pleximeter finger should lie along |
|---|---|

or between, but not across, the ribs. Corresponding zones of the chest should be compared, including the apices, which are assessed by percussing the clavicles directly. Anteriorly, dullness is usually found below the sixth rib, and posteriorly, dullness is usually found at and below the tenth rib. These positions obviously vary with respiration.

*Cardiac dullness*
Loss of cardiac dullness is seen in emphysema, pneumothorax and obesity. Dextrocardia should be remembered as a cause of an apparent loss of cardiac dullness and the opposite side examined.

*Hyperresonance*
*Dullness*
Hyperresonance is a sign of over-inflation as in emphysema while dullness suggests consolidation, lung abscess, atelectasis and fibrosis. Stony dullness is detected over pleural effusions.

Percussion over the sternum may be used to confirm a retrosternal goitre.

*Sternal tenderness*
Percussion of the sternum may elicit tenderness due to marrow proliferation most commonly in acute leukaemia.

---

## AUSCULTATION

**Breath Sounds**
The breath sounds over the upper, middle and lower zones anteriorly, posteriorly and laterally should be listened for using the diaphragm of the stethoscope.

*Vesicular*
Vesicular breath sounds demonstrate an inspiratory phase that is longer than the expiratory phase which follows without a pause; they are soft in character, compared with

*Bronchial*
bronchial breath sounds, which are longer and harsher with a prolonged expiratory phase which follows inspiration after a pause. Bronchial breath sounds are typically heard over consolidation but may also occur with fibrosis and above a pleural effusion.

*Diminished*
Breath sounds are diminished in atelectasis, fibrosis, pneumothorax and absent over a pleural effusion.

## Added sounds

*Crepitations (crackles)*
Crepitations are usually heard during inspiration. They are predominantly fine in early consolidation, medium in pulmonary oedema and coarse in bronchiectasis and fibrosing alveolitis. Crepitations which clear on coughing are not significant.
Crepitations can also be classified by their timing, either as early or late inspiratory: the former due to airways obstruction and the latter in pulmonary oedema, fibrosing alveolitis and sarcoidosis.

*Rhonchi (wheezes)*
Rhonchi are musical blowing sounds which are usually heard in expiration; generalised expiratory rhonchi are characteristic of obstructive airways disease; localised rhonchi suggest focal structural disease.

*Silent chest*
A silent chest in the face of a severe asthmatic attack has a grave prognosis without energetic treatment.

*Pleural rub*
Pleural rubs should be listened for. They are harsh creaking, usually localised sounds, associated with underlying pleural inflammation. Attendant pleuritic chest pain is frequently present.

*Vocal resonance*
Vocal resonance is elicited by asking the patient to repeat the words '111' and '99' whilst listening with the diaphragm of the stethoscope; corresponding areas of each side of the chest should be compared. This provides similar information to tactile vocal fremitus; as before, increased in consolidation and reduced in pleural effusions and collapse.

*Whispering pectoriloquy*
Whispering pectoriloquy is elicited by asking the patient to whisper whilst listening with the diaphragm of the stethoscope; loud transmission of the sound is described as whispering pectoriloquy and may be heard above the fluid level of a pleural effusion and over pneumonic consolidation.

# 8. ABDOMEN

## INSPECTION

### Hands (see Ch. 1)

| | |
|---|---|
| *Finger clubbing* | It is helpful to look briefly at the patient's hands and face before examining the abdomen. In particular, finger clubbing should be looked for as this may occur in association with inflammatory bowel disease and hepatic cirrhosis (see Ch. 1). |
| *Leukonychia*<br>*Koilonychia*<br>*Palmar erythema*<br>*Dupuytren's contracture*<br>*Asterixis*<br>*Tylosis (rare)* | Leukonychia occurs in hypoalbuminaemia and koilonychia in chronic iron deficiency. Palmar erythema, Dupuytren's contracture and flapping tremor (asterixis) should be looked for specifically and, if present, should alert one to look for other stigmata of liver disease. Tylosis of the palms is associated with carcinoma of the oesophagus. |
| *Finger tip atrophy*<br>*Calcinosis* | Atrophy of the finger tips with tightening of the overlying skin and calcinosis is seen in the CRST syndrome (calcinosis, Raynaud's syndrome, sclerodactyly, telangiectasia) which can be associated with an oesophageal motility disturbance. |

### Eyes

| | |
|---|---|
| *Jaundice*<br>*Conjunctival pallor*<br>*Kayser–Fleischer rings (rare)*<br><br>*Xanthelasma* | The sclera should be inspected for jaundice and the conjunctiva for pallor of anaemia. Kayser–Fleischer rings may be seen in hepato-lenticular degeneration (Wilson's disease) as brown rings at the outer corneal margin. Xanthelasma may suggest primary biliary cirrhosis PBC, especially in a jaundiced patient. |

### Face

| | |
|---|---|
| *Cachexia*<br>*Pallor*<br>*Sallow* | A cachectic appearance may suggest an underlying malignancy, whilst pallor occurs in anaemia, and a sallow complexion in renal failure. |

Rhinophyma | Rhinophyma, a complication of acne rosacea, occurs with higher frequency in alcoholic patients.

Parotid swelling | Parotid enlargement due to parotitis may occur in alcohol abuse, Sjögren's syndrome or PBC.

## Mouth

Tongue
Furring | The tongue should be inspected for furring which occurs in patients who breathe through their mouths and is particularly seen in febrile patients and in liver failure and uraemia.

Candidiasis | Candidiasis of the mouth occurs with immunosuppressive therapy, antibiotic use and HIV infection.

Glossitis | Glossitis may occur in iron deficiency anaemia which may complicate gastrointestinal bleeding and may be accompanied by angular cheilitis; it is also seen in the Paterson–Brown Kelly syndrome and in malabsorption states. A painful smooth tongue is seen in pernicious anaemia.

Jaundice | Yellow coloration in the frenulum of the tongue may occur early in hyperbilirubinaemia.

Aphthous ulcers | A small number of patients with aphthous ulceration of the tongue also have inflammatory bowel disease.

Angiomata | Angiomata of the tongue or lips should raise the possibility of hereditary haemorrhagic telangiectasia, especially in patients with gastrointestinal bleeding.

Foetor hepaticus | The sweet musty smell of foetor hepaticus and the distinctive odour of alcohol should be recognised.

## Skin

Many clues may be gained by a brief examination of the skin.

Scratch marks | Jaundice with scratch marks indicates cholestasis.

Pigmentation | Patients with primary biliary cirrhosis are yellow early in the disease but later develop a green-brown colour. Haemochromatosis ('bronzed diabetes') is associated with a slatey-brown pigmentation.

Blisters | In porphyria cutanea tarda, which may be associated with alcoholic liver disease, the skin is fragile and blisters form with slight trauma and in sunlight. In females, this may be associated with hirsutism.

| | |
|---|---|
| *Bruises* | Bruises, in hospital patients, are frequently iatrogenic but do occur more often in those who abuse alcohol and in patients with liver disease. |
| *Tattooing* | An association between tattooing and hepatitis B should be remembered. |
| *Spider naevi* (see Ch. 5) | Normal subjects seldom have more than three spider naevi and the presence of more should alert the examiner to chronic liver disease. Large spider naevi, irrespective of number, should raise the suspicion of liver disease. An increased number of spider naevi is also seen during pregnancy (they disappear within a few months of delivery) and in rheumatoid arthritis. Spider naevi occur mainly in the region of drainage of the superior vena cava, and in particular on the anterior upper chest, neck, face and back of hands. They can be easily differentiated from Campbell de Morgan spots by their capacity to blanch on pressure. |
| *Gynaecomastia* | Gynaecomastia is associated with alcoholic cirrhosis and also with treatment of ascites with spironolactone (see Ch. 7). |
| *Dermatitis* *Dermatitis herpetiformis* | Dermatitis may be associated with vitamin deficiency while dermatitis herpetiformis is associated with coeliac disease. |
| *Pyoderma gangrenosum* | Pyoderma gangrenosum may be seen in inflammatory bowel disease (e.g. ulcerative colitis). A migratory necrolytic erythematous eruption may be seen with a glucagonoma. |
| *Striae* | Striae, which may be red (if recent) or white, occur around the abdomen, shoulders, buttocks and thighs in pregnancy and obesity. In Cushing's syndrome, these striae tend to be purple in colour. |
| **Abdomen** | The abdomen should be inspected both from above and the side. The latter is most easily done by squatting at the patient's bedside. |
| *Shape* | The shape of the abdomen may provide clues to underlying disease. A scaphoid abdomen occurs in starvation, malabsorption and wasting diseases. Abdominal distension, with eversion of the umbilicus, may be due to ascites, which occurs in decompensated cirrhosis, intra-abdominal malignancy, congestive cardiac failure, nephrotic syndrome, peritonitis, constrictive pericarditis, and the Budd–Chiari |
| *Ascites* | |

syndrome. Causes of distension, other than ascites (fluid), include intestinal fluid, obesity (fat), gas (flatus), pregnancy (fetus) and faeces.

*Scars*  Scars should prompt questioning about previous surgical operations.

*Veins*  Dilated, tortuous veins occur in portal hypertension and vena caval obstruction. In portal hypertension, veins tend to radiate from the umbilicus (caput medusa). In inferior vena caval obstruction, venous flow can be demonstrated to be in an upward direction both above and below the umbilicus, whilst in superior vena caval obstruction, the flow is in the opposite direction.

*Discoloration*  Discoloration of the periumbilical area (Cullen's sign) or of the flank (Grey Turner's sign) may be noted with retroperitoneal haemorrhage and in particular in haemorrhagic pancreatitis.

*Hernial orifices*  The hernial orifices must always be inspected for
*Genitalia*  herniae and lymphadenopathy. The genitalia must always be examined in clinical practice. Fistulae and fissures as well as haemorrhoids may be seen in the perianal area.

*Pulsation*  Abdominal pulsations are common in thin individuals but may suggest the presence of an aortic aneurysm. Small intestinal peristalsis may also be seen in thin individuals but will be unduly prominent in intestinal obstruction and their position may give an indication as to the site of obstruction.

*Abdominal wall*  Diminished movement of the abdominal wall
*movement*  muscles is seen in peritonitis.

## PALPATION

**General**  Palpation of areas other than the abdomen is indicated in certain circumstances.
Supraclavicular lymphadenopathy and parotid enlargement should be palpated.

*Tenderness*  After asking the patient to indicate areas of tenderness, which should be examined last, palpation should start lightly, assessing muscle tone and outlining superficial masses. Areas of tenderness should be examined gently, testing for guarding (voluntary muscular contraction) and rebound tenderness. The presence of the latter implies inflammation of the parietal peritoneum. The patient's face must be watched for signs of pain.

*Masses*    The abdomen should then be palpated more deeply to identify intra-abdominal masses. The size, shape, consistency, tenderness, mobility, attachment, fluctuation and associated lymphadenopathy of any mass should be recorded.

**Specific**    Specific examination for enlargement of the liver, spleen, kidneys and bladder should be carried out systematically in the supine patient.

*Liver*    Two main methods of palpating the liver exist. In the most common method, the palpating (right) hand is placed with the index finger lying parallel with the costal margin. Alternatively, the fingers of one or both hands are placed at 90° to the costal margin. In both methods, the liver is felt descending on deep inspiration as controlled firm pressure is applied. The edge is felt with the side of the index finger in the first method and the tips of the fingers using the second. The liver border is palpable in the epigastrium and just below the right costal margin on deep inspiration in normal subjects. Care should be taken not to miss the lower border of a massively enlarged liver in the right iliac fossa.

*Upper border*    Not all livers that are easily palpable are enlarged and the upper border must be determined by percussion to enable the apparently large liver to be differentiated from the displaced low-lying liver in emphysema.

*Riedel's lobe*    A Riedel's lobe, an anatomical variant of the right lobe commoner in females, must be distinguished from hepatomegaly and the right kidney.

*Hepatomegaly*    The commonest causes of hepatomegaly in the UK are cirrhosis, carcinoma and congestive cardiac failure (the 3 C's). Other common causes include fatty liver, myeloproliferative disease and hepatitis (Table 8.1).

*Spleen*    The spleen is a relatively superficial organ and will be missed by too-deep palpation. Examination is bimanual with the left hand placed

**Table 8.1**  Causes of hepatomegaly in UK

| Common | Uncommon |
|---|---|
| Cardiac failure (congestion) | Malaria |
| Carcinoma (metastases, hepatoma, lymphoma) | Polycystic liver |
| Cirrhosis | Riedel's lobe |
| Myeloproliferative disease | Storage diseases (amyloidosis, Gaucher's, Niemann–Pick and glycogen-storage diseases) |
| Viral hepatitis | Budd–Chiari syndrome |
| Fatty liver | Non-viral infections, (TB, hydatid cyst, amoebic abscess, Weil's disease, toxoplasmosis, schistosomiasis) |
| Biliary obstruction | |

postero-laterally over the lower left costal margin with the right hand flat on the abdomen with the fingers pointing towards the left hand. The edge of the spleen descends from under the costal margin in deep inspiration and meets the fingers of the right hand. Examination should begin in the right iliac fossa. The spleen is not felt in health and is only palpable once it has enlarged to 3–4 times its normal size. In situations where the spleen is only just palpable, rolling the patient on to their right side may allow it to be more easily felt. The spleen should be distinguished from the left kidney by five characteristics:

1. it moves freely with respiration
2. you cannot get above the swelling
3. it has a notch on its medial border
4. overlying dullness to percussion
5. a space exists between its posterior edge and erector spinae muscles.

Not all these characteristics are present in all patients.

*Splenomegaly*  The commonest causes of an enlarged spleen in the UK are shown in Table 8.2.

*Kidneys*  The kidneys are frequently not palpable in health, although the lower border of the right kidney may be felt easily in thin patients. Palpation should be bimanual with the left hand posteriorly below the 12th rib and the right hand anteriorly. At the end of deep inspiration, the posterior

**Table 8.2**   Causes of splenomegaly in UK

| Massive | Large | Just Palpable |
|---|---|---|
| Chronic myeloid leukaemia | Portal hypertension | Infective endocarditis |
| Myelofibrosis | Polycythaemia rubra vera | Infectious mononucleosis |
| | Chronic lymphatic leukaemia | |
| | Lymphoma | |
| | Haemolytic anaemias | |
| | Storage disease | |

| | |
|---|---|
| | hand should ballot the kidney onto the deeply palpating right hand. The normal kidney has a characteristic firm and smooth surface. |
| *Renal enlargement* | See Chapter 14. |
| *Adrenal* | Adrenal masses may be palpable and enlarge posteriorly, obliterating the angle between the 12th rib and supra-spinatus muscle. |
| *Bladder* | The bladder is felt arising from the pelvis usually in the midline. In the female, it should be differentiated from a gravid uterus, uterine fibroids and ovarian cysts. |
| *Other masses* | After palpating the abdomen systematically for the above organs, the rest of the abdomen should be carefully palpated. A palpable gallbladder may be noted in the right hypochondrium while an epigastric mass may indicate a gastric carcinoma. The caecum and rectosigmoid colon are often palpable in thin patients; masses in the colon may be neoplastic but should be tested to see if they are indentable (faeces). Uterine and ovarian masses may also be identified. |
| *Fluid thrill* | Where it is indicated (i.e. in patients with abdominal distension) a fluid thrill, if present, should be elicited. A dividing hand over the centre of the abdomen is unnecessary in non-obese patients. |
| *Ballottement/dipping* | When a large volume of ascitic fluid is present, 'dipping' or ballottement may be the only way to identify organomegaly or masses. This is done by rapid depression of the fingertips which, by displacement of fluid, produces a tapping sensation over organs beneath. |

*Succussion splash*   Rocking the patient from side-to-side may
                      produce a succussion splash due to fluid in the
                      stomach. It is only abnormal (indicating gastric
                      stasis or outlet obstruction) if still present 2–3
                      hours postprandially.

*Pulses*              The femoral pulses should routinely be palpated
*Hernial orifices*    at the same time as palpating the hernial orifices.
                      An inguinal hernia originates above the pubic
                      tubercle and may be indirect or direct. A femoral
                      hernia lies in the femoral canal below and lateral
                      to the pubic tubercle. Umbilical, epigastric and
                      incisional hernias may also be noted. All hernias
                      should be examined, their contents identified and
                      their reducibility assessed. A non-reducible
                      hernia which is tender should suggest
                      strangulation.

**Rectal**            The rectal examination is important in clinical
**Examination**       practice and should be performed in all patients.
                      The procedure should first be explained and the
                      patient put on their left side with knees drawn up
                      to the chest. Adequate lubricating jelly on the
                      gloved finger must be used. The anus should be
                      entered slowly and its tone assessed.

*Prostate*            In males, the prostate should be palpated and
                      the median sulcus identified. The texture and size
                      of the gland should be assessed.

*Cervix*              In the female, the cervix and the lateral fornices
                      should be palpated.
                      The remaining three quadrants of the anal canal
                      should be examined in turn, feeling for ulceration,
*Masses*              polyps, masses and tenderness.
                      Remember that piles, unless thrombosed or very
                      large, are seldom palpable. After the finger is
                      withdrawn, the glove should be inspected for
                      blood and faecal occult blood tested for, if
                      indicated.

*Proctoscopy*         If haemorrhoids are suspected proctoscopy is
                      indicated.

**PERCUSSION**        Percussion should be used to confirm both upper
                      and lower borders of the liver and to confirm
                      enlargement of the spleen, as these organs are
                      examined. The upper border of the liver usually

lies at the level of the sixth rib anteriorly. The lower border of the liver should be percussed gently, and always from the area of resonance to the area of dullness. Knowing the upper and lower borders allows estimation of liver size (normal 8–10 cm in mid-clavicular line).

*Shifting dullness*

Percussion is also used to confirm the presence of ascites by eliciting shifting dullness. Once dullness in both flanks has been identified in the supine patient, the line of transition from resonance to dullness should be noted and the patient rolled towards that side whilst keeping the left hand on the line of transition. If fluid is present, the area of dullness will have advanced towards the midline.

*Puddle sign*

The puddle sign of periumbilical dullness to percussion with the patient 'on all fours' can be used to identify small volumes of ascites but is seldom used in clinical practice.

*Bladder size*

Bladder size can be estimated by percussion.

## AUSCULTATION

During the above examination, borborygmi, if audible, should be noted and may indicate intestinal obstruction. They are, however, common in normal subjects.

**Bowel Sounds**

The normal frequency of bowel sounds varies considerably, although more than 30 per minute is usually abnormal and, particularly if loud, suggestive of early intestinal obstruction. Auscultation for at least 30 seconds is necessary before bowel sounds can be declared 'absent'. Diminished or absent bowel sounds occur in peritonitis. In late intestinal obstruction and paralytic ileus, the bowel sounds are high pitched and 'tinkling'.

*Vascular bruit*

Vascular bruits should be listened for specifically, although not all bruits are pathological, especially in the young.

*Vessel-stenosis*

Bruits may arise from stenosis of any intra-abdominal artery, although the site of maximal intensity will help to localise which vessel is involved.

*Hepatic bruit*

Hepatic bruits occur in hepatocellular carcinoma,

alcoholic hepatitis and metastatic lesions. Rarely, a splenic bruit is heard over an enlarged spleen.

*Venous hum*
A loud venous hum at the umbilicus and abdominal wall venous dilatation make up the Cruveilhier–Baumgarten syndrome, usually due to cirrhosis with a congenitally patent umbilical vein. Such a murmur is diagnostically useful in that it implies portal vein patency as the umbilical vein drains into the portal vein.

*Perisplenic rub*
A rub (analogous to pleural rub) may be heard over an area of splenic infarction.

# 9. LEGS

| INSPECTION | The skin of the lower limbs should be inspected. |
|---|---|
| *Atrophy* *Loss of hair* *Pallor* *Gangrene* | Atrophy of the skin is associated with peripheral vascular disease, together with loss of hair, loss of sweating and pale, cold extremities. Cyanosis or gangrene may be seen. Peripheral vascular disease is accelerated in diabetes mellitus when sensory changes may also be present (see Ch. 15). These changes together |
| *Ulceration* | with infection lead to ulceration, which frequently affects pressure points. |
| *Athlete's foot* | Tinea infection of the feet (athlete's foot), seen as flaky lesions between the toes, is common; persistent or extensive infection may be associated with peripheral vascular disease. |
| *Raynaud's phenomenon* | Raynaud's phenomenon causes white, cold, insensitive peripheries followed by cyanosis and then redness. If severe, atrophic changes may occur with time. Causes include connective tissue diseases, cryoglobulinaemia, drugs (ergotamine) and idiopathic. |
| *Oedema* | Ankle oedema should be looked for specifically. If present, a check should be made to see if pitting on pressure occurs. The pressure must be applied for at least 5 seconds over a bony landmark, usually the lower tibia. Pitting oedema is usually due to congestive cardiac failure, hypoalbuminaemia or venous insufficiency. |
| *Lymphoedema* | Painless swelling of the legs occurs in lymphoedema which affects mainly the dorsal aspect of the feet and toes, is brawny in colour and pits poorly on pressure. It can occur in Milroy's disease in women, neoplasia and elephantiasis. |
| *Varicose veins* *Stasis dermatitis* | Varicose veins may be seen together with stasis dermatitis or ulceration above and behind the medial malleoli. |

| | |
|---|---|
| Ulceration | Ulceration of the legs also may be associated with peripheral vascular disease, diabetes, neuropathy (e.g. due to alcohol, tabes, syringomyelia), infection, haemolytic anaemia, connective tissue diseases, trauma and neoplasia. |
| Deep vein thrombosis | Swelling of the leg with oedema, redness or duskiness and dilated superficial veins may be seen in deep venous thrombosis; a ruptured |
| Baker's cyst | Baker's cyst can cause similar changes in the calf. Frequently, deep venous thromboses are clinically silent. |
| Pyoderma gangrenosum | See Chapter 8. |
| Necrobiosis lipoidica | The raised red lesions with necrotic centres of necrobiosis lipoidica may be seen in diabetes. |
| Pretibial myxoedema | The mauve-coloured pretibial swelling of pretibial myxoedema may be seen in hyperthyroidism. |
| Erythema nodosum | Raised erythematous discrete nodules of erythema nodosum may be seen with drug sensitivity (penicillin, sulphonamides), streptococcal and mycoplasmal infections, tuberculosis, leprosy, sarcoidosis, rheumatoid arthritis, rheumatic fever, ulcerative colitis and systemic fungal infections. |
| Vasculitis | Palpable purpuric spots with necrotic centres may be seen with vasculitis in connective tissue diseases and meningococcal septicaemia. |
| Purpura | Purpura may first be noted in the legs and occurs when platelet defects are present, whilst |
| Ecchymoses | ecchymoses suggest a coagulopathy or endothelial fragility (e.g. scurvy). |
| Keratoderma blenorrhagica | See Chapter 21. |
| Toe clubbing | Clubbing of the toes may occur in some patients with finger clubbing and carries the same significance. |
| Muscle wasting | The musculature should be inspected for wasting. This is generalised in cachexia, but proximal in osteomalacia, limb-girdle dystrophy, thyroid disease, Cushing's syndrome, and diabetic amyotrophy. Distal wasting is seen in peripheral neuropathies such as peroneal muscle atrophy, whilst localised muscle wasting is typical of peripheral nerve lesions. Wasting and deformity of one leg may suggest old poliomyelitis. |

| | |
|---|---|
| *Length* | If one leg appears to be shortened, the true length of each leg should be measured from the anterior superior iliac spine to the medial malleolus. Apparent shortening, due to pelvic tilt, will then become obvious. |
| *Foot drop* | Foot drop may be due to lateral popliteal nerve damage, prolapsed intervertebral disc, polyneuropathy or simply prolonged bed-rest. |
| *Fasciculation* | Fasciculation may be noted in lower motor neurone lesions as occurs in amyotrophic lateral sclerosis, cervical spondylosis, syringomyelia and root compression due to prolapse of a lumbar intervertebral disc. |
| *Abnormal movements/posture* | Inspect for abnormal movements — athetosis, tremor or spasm, and postural abnormalities (e.g. pes cavus, genu valgum or varum, and internal or external rotation). |

## PALPATION

| | |
|---|---|
| *Arterial pulses* | The main arterial pulses in the legs should be checked (i.e. femoral, popliteal, posterior tibial and dorsalis pedis). |
| *Temperature* | Cold peripheries occur with both arterial and venous insufficiency. Deep venous thrombosis is associated with an increased temperature in the affected leg which is usually also tender. The leg circumference should be measured if one leg appears swollen or wasted. |
| *Superficial thrombophlebitis* | The tender, warm, red, palpable thrombosed veins of superficial thrombophlebitis should be noted if present. |
| *Varicose veins* | Varicose veins can be tested by Trendelenberg test, i.e. elevate the leg then apply pressure over the origin of the long saphenous vein. If the patient then stands up and the veins do not fill, the long saphenous vein is competent. |
| *Femoral triangle* | Tenderness may be elicited in the femoral triangle when a deep venous thrombosis is present there. |
| *Joints* | Examination of joints is outlined in Chapter 21. |
| **Tone** | Tone should be assessed in a relaxed patient. Rolling the leg back and forth on the bed may give some idea of tone. However, the hip, knee |

| | and ankle should be put through a full range of passive movements for tone to be fully assessed. |
|---|---|
| *Hypotonia* | Hypotonia occurs in lower motor neurone lesions and acute upper motor neurone lesions, whilst |
| *Spasticity* | hypertonia with spasticity (clasp knife) is seen in established upper motor neurone lesions. |
| *Plastic rigidity* *'Cog-wheeling'* | Plastic (lead-pipe) rigidity occurs in parkinsonism with 'cog-wheeling' when a superimposed tremor is present. |

**Power**  Power should be tested in the muscle groups shown in Table 9.1.

In lower motor neurone lesions diminished power is associated with flaccid wasted muscles and fasciculation, whilst in upper motor neurone lesions diminished power coexists with increased tone, minor muscle wasting and clonus.

**Coordination**  See Chapter 19.

**Gait**  Certain typical gait patterns are described in Table 9.2.

**Reflexes**  The knee (L3,4) and ankle jerks (L5,S1) should be elicited and clonus looked for if hyperreflexia is present.

*Hyporeflexia*  Hyporeflexia occurs in lower motor neurone lesions, myopathies and with acute upper motor neurone damage.

**Table 9.1**  Muscle group for power testing

| Group | Roots |
|---|---|
| Hip flexion | L1,2,3 (iliopsoas) |
| Hip extension | L5 (glutei) |
| Knee extension | L3,4 (quadriceps) |
| Knee flexion | L5,S1 (hamstrings) |
| Ankle dorsiflexion | L4,5 |
| Ankle plantar flexion | S1,2 (gastrocnemius) |
| Ankle inversion | L4 (ant. & post. tibial) |
| Ankle eversion | L5,S1 (peronei) |
| Toe extension | L5,S1 |
| Toe flexion | S2,3 |

**Table 9.2**  Some typical gait patterns

| Gait | Pattern | Cause |
|------|---------|-------|
| Hemiplegic | Extended leg, flexed arm Pelvis tilts to allow affected leg round and forward | Cerebrovascular accident |
| Paraparetic (Scissor) | Stiffness of both legs Feet remain on ground | Cerebral palsy, cord compression, multiple sclerosis, syringomyelia |
| Cerebellar | Wide-based, reeling, unsteady, staggering towards lesion | Cerebellar lesions, multiple sclerosis, alcoholism, myxoedema |
| Festinating | Rigidity, shuffling, festination with stooped posture | Parkinsonism |
| Waddling | Hips tilted alternately (glutei weak) | Congenital dislocation of the hips Proximal myopathy Limb-girdle dystrophy Old polio |
| Steppage | Foot drop, high lift, slaps on floor | Lateral popliteal nerve palsy Peroneal muscular atrophy |
| Stamping | High stepping, wide base, stamps (loss of position sense) | $B_{12}$ deficiency, tabes dorsalis, diabetes mellitus |
| Marche à petit pas | Small steps Stooped posture | Parkinsonism |
| Astasia-abasia | Tendency to fall backwards | Elderly, frontal lobe lesion |

*Absent jerks*      Retest with reinforcement before saying reflexes are absent.

*Hyperreflexia*      Hyperreflexia occurs in upper motor neurone lesions, thyrotoxicosis, hepatic coma and uraemia.

*Pendular jerks*      Pendular reflex jerks occur with cerebellar

*Slow relaxation*      lesions, whilst a slow relaxation phase is typical in hypothyroidism.

*Plantar reflex*      The plantar reflex (L5,S1), elicited by stroking the lateral border of the sole of the foot, is flexor in normal subjects and extensor (Babinski's sign) in upper motor neurone lesions. A fresh orange stick is probably best used for this test in each patient.

*Oppenheim's test*      Oppenheim's test is an equivalent test and is elicited by applying pressure along the anterior surface of the tibia.

*Rossolimo's sign*      Rossolimo's sign, elicited by flicking the distal phalanges of the toes in an extensor direction,

produces brisk plantar flexion of the great toe in
upper motor neurone lesions. Absent knee and
ankle jerks, associated with an extensor plantar
reflex, are seen in tabes dorsalis, subacute
combined degeneration of cord, diabetic
neuropathy, motor neurone disease and
Friedreich's ataxia.

## Other Signs

*Kernig's sign*

Kernig's sign, elicited by flexing the hip and knee
followed by knee extension, produces hamstring
spasm in meningism. Associated signs such as
neck stiffness and photophobia should be
elicited.

*Straight leg raising
test*

A prolapsed intervertebral disc at L5/S1
produces pain in the back of the leg if the hip is
flexed with the knee extended (the straight leg
raising test).

*Femoral nerve
stretch test*

Prolapse of the intervertebral disc at L2/3
produces pain in the back if the knee is flexed in
a prone patient with extended hips (the femoral
nerve stretch test).

## Sensation

*Light touch
Pin prick
Temperature*

Check sensation using both light touch and pin
prick. Temperature sensation should only be
tested in certain patients. Remember the
dermatomes: L1 — inguinal area; L2,3 — anterior
thigh; L4,5 — shin; S1 — lateral border foot, sole,
back of calf.

*Vibration*

Vibration should be tested with a low frequency
(128 Hz) tuning fork on the malleoli, patellae and
anterior superior iliac spines. Position sense
should be tested by either wiggling the toes,
initially very gently with a gradually increasing arc
and asking when the movement is felt, or by the
conventional method of asking the patient to
identify upward and downward movements.
Loss of sensation is symmetrical and distal in
neuropathy due to diabetes mellitus, thiamine
deficiency, carcinomatous neuropathy and drugs.
Dorsal column damage produces vibration sense
loss (without spinothalamic loss) in both legs in
vitamin $B_{12}$ deficiency and tabes dorsalis and in
the ipsi-lateral leg in the Brown–Sequard

| | syndrome (where the contralateral leg has spinothalamic loss). |
|---|---|
| *Sensory inattention* | The inability to discriminate the fact that both legs are being touched at once while each leg is correctly identified when touched separately is sensory inattention and is seen with parietal lobe lesions particularly of the non-dominant cerebral hemisphere. |

# 10. ANAEMIA

Not all pale looking patients are anaemic, whilst even severe anaemia may be missed clinically unless specifically looked for. As well as identifying the presence of anaemia, examination may provide important clues as to its aetiology and effects.

## INSPECTION

### General

*Pallor*

*Palmar creases*
*Mucous membranes*

*Cachexia*

Generalised pallor may suggest anaemia (Table 10.1), but other causes of pallor such as shock and panhypopituitarism should be borne in mind. Pallor of skin creases of the hands should be present as well as pallor of the mucous membranes (mouth, conjunctivae) before concluding that a patient is anaemic.
The cause of anaemia may be suggested from the general appearance — the cachexia of cancer, the archetypal white hair, blue eyes and

**Table 10.1**   Physical signs in common anaemias

| Iron deficiency | $B_{12}$ deficiency | Underlying neoplasm |
| --- | --- | --- |
| Pallor | Pallor | Pallor |
| CVS signs | CVS signs | CVS signs |
| Koilonychia | Jaundice | Palpable tumour |
| Glossitis | Premature greying | Cachexia |
| Angular cheilitis | Glossitis, glossodynia | Clubbing |
| | Subacute combined degeneration of the cord | Lymphadenopathy |
| | | Often also signs of iron deficiency |

| | |
|---|---|
| *Pernicious anaemia* | lemon tinge to the skin of pernicious anaemia, |
| *Pregnancy* | and pregnancy (folate and iron deficiency). |
| *Racial origin* | The racial origin of the patient should be noted. Haemoglobinopathies are commoner in Negroes and Asiatics, while thalassaemia is commoner around the Mediterranean coast and the Far East. |
| *Stature* | Shortness of stature occurs with the hereditary anaemias. |
| *Oedema* | Ankle oedema should be looked for and may indicate right heart failure secondary to anaemia. |

**Skin** — Apart from pallor, characteristic changes occur in certain specific anaemias.

| | |
|---|---|
| *Jaundice* | Jaundice occurs in haemolytic anaemias, neoplastic invasion of the liver, and chronic liver |
| *Uraemia* | disease, whilst in uraemia a muddy complexion is characteristic. |
| *Hypothyroidism* | The features of hypothyroidism are described in Chapter 2. |
| *Ecchymoses* | Ecchymoses may be present, suggesting a coagulopathy or scurvy. In the latter there may be perifollicular haemorrhages. |
| *Petechiae* | Petechiae suggest a platelet production problem such as autoimmune thrombocytopenia, aplastic anaemia, leukaemia, lymphoma or secondary replacement of the marrow with cancer. The Hess test, where a sphygmomanometer cuff is inflated to the mid-way point between systolic and diastolic pressures for 5 minutes, may disclose a petechial tendency. |
| *Dermatitis* | An exfoliative dermatitis may mean an underlying lymphoma. |
| *Psoriasis* | Severe psoriasis may be treated with methotrexate causing a secondary folate deficiency anaemia. |
| *Scars* | Scars of abdominal surgery might suggest 'post-gastrectomy' or ileal resection as a cause of anaemia ($B_{12}$ ± iron deficiency). |

**Nails**

| | |
|---|---|
| *Brittleness* | Iron deficiency causes brittle nails and |
| *Koilonychia* | koilonychia, a characteristic spoon-shaped deformity. |
| *Clubbing* | Clubbing of the nails may be associated with anaemia in malabsorption states, ulcerative colitis, carcinoma or infective endocarditis. |

| | |
|---|---|
| *Splinter haemorrhages* | Infective endocarditis may also give rise to splinter haemorrhages. |
| *Lindsay's nails* | Chronic renal failure may be associated with Lindsay's nails — pallor of the nails with a distal brown arc. |

## Hands

| | |
|---|---|
| *Rheumatoid arthritis* *Osteoarthrosis* | Examination of the hands may reveal typical changes of rheumatoid arthritis or osteoarthrosis. In the former, the primary disease state may contribute to the anaemia, while in both diseases the treatment may cause anaemia (e.g. anti-inflammatory drugs causing gastrointestinal blood loss). |
| *Dactylitis* | Dactylitis, seen as a swollen and often tender finger, occurs in some haemoglobinopathies, especially sickle-cell disease as well as syphilis, sarcoidosis and tuberculosis. |

## Eyes

Conjunctival pallor should be looked for as should icterus. Conjunctival haemorrhages may be seen in leukaemia. Fundal changes which may occur are mentioned in Chapter 3.

## Mouth/Tongue

| | |
|---|---|
| *Glossitis* | Atrophic glossitis, a smooth, red and often painful tongue, occurs in iron, vitamin $B_{12}$ and folic acid deficiency anaemias. |

## Mucous Membranes

Pallor is common to all anaemias.

| | |
|---|---|
| *Telangiectases* | Small telangiectases may be seen in the mouth as well as on the skin in hereditary haemorrhagic telangiectasia. |
| *Cheilitis* | Cracking and soreness of the angle of the lips, angular cheilitis, is seen in iron and B vitamin deficiencies and with ill-fitting dentures. |

## Gums

| | |
|---|---|
| *Hypertrophy* | Hypertrophy of the gums is seen with chronic phenytoin use which may cause folate deficiency. Hypertrophy with bleeding and infection is seen in the rare acute monocytic leukaemia. |

| | |
|---|---|
| *Blue lines* | Blue lines occur in lead poisoning which causes haemolytic anaemia and is a marrow toxin. |
| *Bleeding* | Bleeding from the gums is seen in scurvy and in thrombocytopenia but only if the patient has teeth. The association of swollen bleeding gums |
| *Vincent's angina* | with halitosis should suggest Vincent's angina. |
| **Pharynx** | Ulceration of the pharynx and tonsillar swelling may be seen in leukaemia, lymphoma or aplastic anaemia. |

## PALPATION

| | |
|---|---|
| *Pulse* | The pulse rate and volume should be recorded and may provide information regarding the severity of the anaemia. |
| *Lymphadenopathy* | Localised lymphadenopathy may accompany a primary neoplasm such as Troissier's sign (left supraclavicular (Virchow's) node swelling in gastric carcinoma), while generalised lymphadenopathy would favour lymphoma or chronic lymphatic leukaemia. The lymph nodes involved by lymphoma are frequently rubbery in nature in distinction to the hard craggy nodes of metastatic carcinoma. |
| **Abdomen** | Tenderness in the epigastrium may occur in peptic ulcer disease. |
| *Hepatomegaly* | Hepatomegaly can occur in alcohol-related chronic liver disease which is also associated with poor diet, iron metabolism problems, folate deficiency or gastric bleeding. It may also occur in congestive cardiac failure secondary to anaemia. |
| *Splenomegaly* | Splenomegaly is massive in chronic myeloid leukaemia and myelofibrosis; moderate or just palpable in lymphomas, portal hypertension, haemolytic anaemias (except sickle-cell) and pernicious anaemia. |
| *Kidneys* | Large polycystic kidneys may be palpable and be responsible for renal failure. |
| *Masses* | A palpable mass may suggest an underlying malignancy of the stomach or colon. |
| *Rectal* | Rectal examination may reveal melaena, faeces positive for occult blood, haemorrhoids or tumour. |

| | |
|---|---|
| *Pelvis* | Pelvic examination may reveal the cause of menorrhagia. |

## CNS

| | |
|---|---|
| *Subacute combined degeneration* | Subacute combined degeneration of the cord may accompany pernicious anaemia and is identified by loss of vibration and position sense of the lower limbs, together with a 'glove-and-stocking' sensory loss. Ankle and knee jerks may also be lost. |
| *Lead poisoning* | Lead poisoning may cause a distal motor neuropathy. |
| *Meningism* | Meningism may be seen in acute leukaemias if there is CNS involvement. |

## PERCUSSION

Percussion is of limited use in assessing a patient with anaemia but sternal or vertebral tenderness may be present in neoplastic disease.

## AUSCULTATION

| | |
|---|---|
| *Heart murmurs* | Auscultation of the heart may reveal 'flow' murmurs which resolve once the anaemia is treated. Heart murmurs associated with anaemia |
| *Blood pressure* | occur in infective endocarditis. The blood pressure should always be recorded and frequently shows a wide pulse pressure in anaemic patients. The presence of a postural drop in particular should raise the possibility of an actively bleeding lesion. |

# 11. POLYCYTHAEMIA

Examination of patients with polycythaemia may indicate the cause and may also show complications of the condition. Polycythaemia is defined as a raised red cell mass ($>6 \times 10^6$ RBC/ml or haematocrit $>0.55$) and is due to increased production of red cells. This may be primarily due to increased marrow production (polycythaemia rubra vera) or secondary to hypoxia — high altitude, haemoglobinopathies, cyanotic congenital heart disease, chronic obstructive airways disease, renal disease (cysts and tumours), uterine fibroids, hepatoma and cerebellar haemangioblastoma. Spurious polycythaemia (due to relative high red cell mass with a low plasma volume) is associated with smoking, anxiety and hypertension.

## INSPECTION

### General

| | |
|---|---|
| *Plethora* | Facial plethora is often noted in polycythaemia. |
| *Cyanosis* | Cyanosis (due to desaturation of more than 5 g/l haemoglobin may also be present). |
| | Central cyanosis occurs in cyanotic congenital heart disease and chronic obstructive airways |
| *Conjunctival injection* | disease. Conjunctival injection may also be present. |
| *Tar staining* | Tar staining of fingers is common in smokers, who may have chronic obstructive airways disease or spurious polycythaemia (due to decreased plasma volume). |
| *Clubbing* | Clubbing of fingernails may be seen in cyanotic congenital heart disease and bronchial carcinoma. |

| | |
|---|---|
| *Gout* | Gouty tophi and hot, tender, swollen, red joints of gout may complicate primary polycythaemia. |
| *Obesity* | Marked obesity associated with somnolence, due to hypoventilation, may give rise to secondary polycythaemia in the Pickwickian syndrome. |

**Chest**  Tachypnoea and dyspnoea may be noted in patients with chronic obstructive airways disease who will also have diminished chest expansion. Cyanotic congenital heart disease may have other clinical signs (see Ch. 6).

**Legs**

| | |
|---|---|
| *PVD* | Signs of peripheral vascular disease — white, cold legs with diminished sweating, atrophic skin with loss of hair and perhaps ulceration and gangrene — may be noted and are due to the hyperviscosity associated with polycythaemia. |
| *DVT* | Polycythaemia also predisposes to deep venous thrombosis (hot, swollen, tender calf with bluish discoloration and distended superficial veins). |

---

## PALPATION

### Abdomen

| | |
|---|---|
| *Hepatosplenomegaly* | Hepatosplenomegaly is often found in primary polycythaemia while hepatomegaly alone may be due to hepatoma. |
| *Large kidneys* | Large kidneys may be due to hydronephrosis, renal cysts, polycystic disease and renal adenocarcinoma (hypernephroma). |
| *Uterine fibroids* | Giant uterine fibroids may cause polycythaemia. |
| *Rectal examination* | Faeces positive for occult blood obtained at rectal examination may reflect the higher incidence of gastrointestinal haemorrhage in polycythaemia. |

---

## CNS

| | |
|---|---|
| *Cerebellar signs* | Examination of the CNS may reveal cerebellar signs associated with cerebellar haemangioblastoma — ipsilateral ataxia, |

incoordination, nystagmus, hypotonia, pendular tendon jerks, pass-pointing, dysdiadochokinesia (see Ch. 19). It may also reveal signs of a cerebrovascular accident (hemiplegia with increased tone, hyperreflexia and hemianopia). Cerebral thrombosis may complicate polycythaemia.

*Fundal examination*   Engorged retinal veins with a dark background may be seen.

## PERCUSSION

Percussion may be used to demonstrate hyperresonance in an emphysematous chest and is useful in confirming organomegaly on abdominal examination.

## AUSCULTATION

*Bruits*   Arterial bruits may be present in patients with peripheral or cerebral vascular disease. A bruit may also be heard over a hepatoma.

*Blood pressure*   Hypertension is common in primary polycythaemia, and spurious polycythaemia is associated with hypertension and anxiety (Gaisbock's syndrome).

# 12. CYANOSIS

Patients with suspected cyanosis must be examined in good, natural light. The blue discoloration of cyanosis is due to an excess of reduced haemoglobin in the capillaries. Over 5 g/dl of haemoglobin must be present before cyanosis is apparent (i.e. approximately less than 85% saturated or $PaO_2$ less than 60 mmHg (8.0 K Pascal)). Cyanosis must be classified as peripheral or central.

**Peripheral Cyanosis**

Peripheral cyanosis is due to low cardiac output, peripheral vascular disease, increased tissue oxygen extraction and extreme cold weather.

**Central Cyanosis**

Central cyanosis is due to inadequate oxygenation of the blood; causes include acute and chronic lung disease, pulmonary embolism, hypoventilation, decrease in inspired oxygen, polycythaemia, and right-to-left cardiac shunts.

**Differential Cyanosis**

Differential cyanosis with normal upper limbs and cyanosed lower limbs occurs with reversal of the shunt across a patent ductus arteriosus.

## INSPECTION

**Face**

*Buccal mucosa*
*Tongue*
*Lips*

In central cyanosis there is always cyanosis at the periphery but the distinguishing feature is cyanosis of the buccal mucosa, tongue and lips.

**Hands**

In peripheral cyanosis the hands are cold and blue, as are other exposed parts.

*Clubbing*

Clubbing of the fingers is seen in cyanotic

congenital heart disease and fibrotic lung disease (see Ch. 1).

*Flapping tremor*  A flapping tremor in an acute exacerbation of chronic bronchitis or emphysema reflects carbon dioxide retention (see Ch.1), while a fine tremor may reflect the use of sympathomimetic bronchodilators in these conditions.

## Legs

*Venous stasis*  Poor venous drainage with stasis results in cyanosis and can be assessed by the time it takes for veins to empty on elevating the leg;

*Ankle oedema*  ankle oedema is frequently found in this condition.

*DVT*  Signs of deep venous thrombosis may or may not be seen in association with a pulmonary embolus.

## Neck

*Elevated JVP*  The jugular venous pressure may be elevated in cor pulmonale, pulmonary hypertension or pulmonary embolism.

*Accessory muscles*  Accessory muscles of respiration are frequently used in chronic bronchitis and emphysema.

*Trachea*  Shortening of the crico-sternal distance (see Ch. 7) occurs in obstructive airways disease.

**Chest**  Hypoventilation with a slow respiratory rate may cause central cyanosis and this may occur with cerebrovascular accidents and with drug overdosage.

*Dyspnoea*
*Tachypnoea*  Dyspnoea with a fast respiratory rate may occur in acute exacerbations of chronic bronchitis and emphysema, pulmonary thromboembolism and sometimes in cyanotic congenital heart disease.

*Barrel chest*
*Pigeon chest*  Barrel chest deformity is associated with chronic bronchitis and emphysema while a pigeon chest is sometimes seen in cyanotic congenital heart disease.

## PALPATION

### Pulse

*Peripheral pulses*  Peripheral pulses may be weak or absent in

| | peripheral vascular disease and should be checked routinely. |
|---|---|
| *Tachycardia* | A tachycardia may be associated with bronchodilator use and occurs after a pulmonary thromboembolism and in left ventricular failure, often with a gallop rhythm. |

## Chest

| *Diminished expansion* | Diminished chest expansion occurs in chronic bronchitis and emphysema. |
|---|---|
| *Right ventricular heave* | A right ventricular heave may be palpable in cor pulmonale and in cyanotic congenital heart disease and the latter may be associated with a thrill. |

## Abdomen

| *Hepatosplenomegaly* *Hepatomegaly* | Hepatosplenomegaly may be evident in polycythaemia rubra vera, while hepatomegaly is common in congestive cardiac failure. |
|---|---|

## PERCUSSION

| | Percussion of the chest may reveal |
|---|---|
| *Hyperresonance* *Stony dullness* | hyperresonance with emphysema, dullness in pneumonic consolidation or stony dullness with a pleural effusion in, for example, pulmonary thromboembolism or bronchial carcinoma. |

## AUSCULTATION

### Lungs

| *Rhonchi* *Crepitations* | Auscultation of the chest may reveal rhonchi or wheeze in chronic bronchitis and early inspiratory crepitations due to small airway obstruction. Late inspiratory crepitations may be due to pulmonary congestion in left ventricular failure and cyanotic congenital heart disease or fibrosis, as in idiopathic fibrosing alveolitis. Bronchial breathing and crepitations may be heard over pneumonic consolidation. |
|---|---|
| *Pleural rub* | A pleural rub may be heard with pneumonia or pulmonary thromboembolism. |

## Heart

*Pulmonary systolic murmur*

Congenital heart disease can be divided into cyanotic and acyanotic varieties. In the cyanotic type, a right-to-left shunt exists. This group includes Fallot's tetralogy, Eisenmegner's complex and transposition of the great vessels. Murmurs appropriate for these conditions should be listened for carefully.

**False Cyanosis**

Blue discoloration which simulates cyanosis occurs in methaemoglobinaemia and sulphaemoglobinaemia which are usually drug related.

# 13. JAUNDICE

The commonest causes of jaundice in the United Kingdom, which should be borne in mind when examining an icteric patient, are hepatitis, cirrhosis, gallstones, pancreatic carcinoma, hepatic congestion, drugs and Gilbert's disease. Clues to the aetiology should be sought.

## INSPECTION

### General

| | |
|---|---|
| *Jaundice* | The presence of jaundice should be confirmed by inspecting, in good natural lighting, the sclera and skin. The frenulum of the tongue may exhibit a yellow discoloration early in hyperbilirubinaemia. |
| *Carotenaemia* | Yellow skin with white sclera may be seen in carotenaemia such as occurs in hypothyroidism or food faddists (obsessional carrot eaters). Hyperbilirubinaemia can be detected clinically as jaundice only once it has reached approximately 50 μmol/l. The severity of jaundice should be gauged. A greenish tinge due to biliverdin deposition suggests chronic jaundice as may occur in primary biliary cirrhosis or chronic extrahepatic biliary obstruction. |
| *Pigmentation* | Other abnormalities of pigmentation as well as jaundice may be present in patients with liver disease, such as the slatey-grey complexion in haemochromatosis, areas of patchy, hyper- and hypopigmentation in porphyria cutanea tarda, and vitiligo in chronic active hepatitis and pernicious anaemia. |
| *Grey complexion* | |
| *Patchy, hyper- and hypopigmentation* | |
| *Vitiligo* | |
| *Acanthosis nigricans* | Acanthosis nigricans, a brownish, thickened, velvety area of skin, especially on the back of |

the neck, in the axillae, perianally or in the inguinal region, in adults is associated with malignancy, particularly pancreatic.

*Pseudo-acanthosis nigricans*
Pseudo-acanthosis nigricans occurs in diabetes mellitus, polycystic ovary syndrome and obesity.

*Scratch marks*
Cholestatic jaundice frequently produces pruritus, possibly due to skin deposition of bile acids. Scratch marks therefore should be sought.

*Injection marks*
Evidence of intravenous drug abuse should be looked for and, if found, should alert one to the possibility of hepatitis B and HIV infection.

*Weight loss*
Evidence of recent weight loss may be seen in patients with liver disease and/or malignancy.

## Head and Neck

*Cushingoid facies*
A Cushingoid appearance may occur in alcohol abuse or be due to steroid therapy used to treat such conditions as chronic active hepatitis.

*Xanthelasma*
The lids and periorbital tissue should be inspected for xanthelasmata which are

*Kayser–Fleischer rings (rare)*
associated with chronic cholestasis, and the eyes for Kayser–Fleischer rings of Wilson's disease.

*Anaemia*
The combination of anaemia and jaundice occurs with haemolysis and with gastrointestinal bleeding associated with cirrhosis or with gastrointestinal malignancy with hepatic metastases.

Examination of the remainder of the face may reveal some clues as to the cause of jaundice. The alcohol abuser frequently has a flushed appearance with or without other clues such as

*Acne rosacea*
*Rhinophyma*
*Parotitis*
acne rosacea, rhinophyma, paper-money telangiectasis, parotitis and spider naevi (see Ch. 5).

*JVP*
A raised jugular venous pressure should be looked for as it may occur secondary to a pericardial effusion due to malignancy or with hypoalbuminaemia or in congestive cardiac failure which may cause such hepatic congestion as to cause jaundice.

*Breath*
The breath should be smelt for the sickly sweet odour of hepatic foetor.

## Limbs

*Leukonychia*
The hands should be examined for leukonychia,

| | |
|---|---|
| *Finger clubbing* *Palmar erythema* *Dupuytren's contracture* *Asterixis* | finger clubbing, palmar erythema, Dupuytren's contracture and asterixis, all of which occur in liver disease. |
| *Smooth nails* | Shiny smooth nails may be produced by repeated scratching. |
| *Ankle oedema* | Ankle oedema should be checked for and, if present, may suggest either hypoalbuminaemia or congestive cardiac failure. |
| *Pyoderma gangrenosum* | Pyoderma gangrenosum or erythema nodosum should alert one to the possibility of sclerosing cholangitis secondary to inflammatory bowel disease. |
| *Thrombophlebitis* | Thrombophlebitis is associated with pancreatic carcinoma. |

## Trunk

| | |
|---|---|
| *Gynaecomastia* *Spider naevi* *Venous distension* *Ascites* | The chest and abdomen should be inspected for gynaecomastia, spider naevi, venous distension, including the rare caput medusae, and the flank distension and umbilical herniation produced by ascites. |
| *Reduced body hair* | Absent or diminished axillary and pubic hair should be looked for as a stigma of chronic liver disease. |
| *Masses* | Large abdominal masses may be visible as may cutaneous metastases. |
| *Surgical scars* | Scars of previous surgery should be identified and interpreted. A recent cholecystectomy suggests retained common bile duct stones as a cause of jaundice. Any recent surgery raises the possibility of halothane hepatitis. This usually follows exposure to multiple anaesthetics. Blood transfusions used peri-operatively may have caused infective hepatitis. |
| *Ileostomy* | The presence of an ileostomy in a jaundiced patient should suggest sclerosing cholangitis complicating ulcerative colitis or hepatic metastases after resection of a colonic carcinoma. |

## PALPATION

| | |
|---|---|
| *Lymphadenopathy* | Lymphadenopathy in the jaundiced patient occurs in infectious mononucleosis, lymphoma and other |

malignancies and should be identified by palpation of cervical, supraclavicular, axillary and groin lymph nodes.

*Gynaecomastia*    Gynaecomastia should be confirmed by identifying palpable breast tissue rather than fat.

*Breast lumps*    In females, the breasts, the commonest site of primary malignancy, should always be examined.

## Abdomen

*Liver size/shape/ tenderness*    The abdomen should be palpated carefully, paying particular attention to liver size, shape, texture, pulsatility and tenderness. Remember that cirrhotic livers may be small and non-palpable. A tender liver edge suggests hepatitis or congestion; a hard, non-tender edge with splenomegaly, cirrhosis and an irregular outline suggests metastases. Tenderness below the costal margin at the ninth rib anteriorly is associated with cholecystitis (Murphy's sign) but is not specific for gallbladder inflammation.

*Gallbladder*    The gallbladder should be palpated for as a cystic swelling in the right hypochondrium and if identified implies obstruction of the bile duct beyond entry of the cystic duct. Although the presence of a palpable gallbladder in a jaundiced patient is said to exclude gallstones as the cause (Courvoisier's law), it should also be remembered that an enlarged gallbladder is frequently missed on examination.

*Choledochal cyst*    A mass in the epigastrium in a young female with jaundice should alert the examiner to the possibility of a choledochal cyst, which affects females four times more often than males.

*Pancreas*    Occasionally a pancreatic carcinoma or pseudo-cyst will be palpable in the epigastrium.

*Spleen*    The spleen, if palpable, suggests cirrhosis, haemolytic anaemia, hereditary spherocytosis, lymphoma or infectious mononucleosis.

*Genitalia*    In practice, the genitalia should be examined for testicular atrophy, associated with chronic alcoholism or enlargement due to neoplasm which might also involve the liver (teratoma, lymphoma).

*Rectal examination*    In practice, a rectal examination is essential in the complete examination of the jaundiced patient.

## PERCUSSION

| | |
|---|---|
| *Masses* | Percussion should be used to confirm enlargement of organs and the presence of masses or ascites. Percuss the lower and upper borders of the liver, moving up from below, down from above. Demonstrate the liver span in the mid-clavicular line and identify the interspace of its upper border. |
| *Ascites* | Ascites in a jaundiced patient is compatible with malignancy, cirrhosis or severe right ventricular failure. |
| *Lung fields* | Percussion over the lungs should be carried out to detect areas of consolidation or effusion related to lung tumours. |

## AUSCULTATION

| | |
|---|---|
| *Hepatic bruit* | A bruit over the liver occurs in hepatitis and primary or secondary liver tumours, all of which may cause jaundice. |
| *Lung fields* | Auscultation over the lung fields should be performed especially if abnormalities are detected on percussion or malignancy is a strong possibility. |
| **Faeces** **Urine** | Examination of the jaundiced patient is incomplete without examining the colour of the stools and testing the urine for urobilinogen and conjugated bilirubin. It should be remembered that urobilinogen is colourless in fresh urine. |

# 14. URAEMIA

Uraemia frequently develops incipiently and should always be considered when examining patients complaining of general malaise. Thorough examination may provide important clues as to the underlying disease process. The commonest causes of chronic renal failure in the UK are chronic glomerulonephritis, chronic pyelonephritis, diabetes mellitus and hypertension.

## INSPECTION

### General

| | |
|---|---|
| *Conscious level* | The conscious level of the patient should be assessed and drowsiness, a common feature of advanced renal failure, noted. |
| *Respiration* | The type and rate of respiration should be noted. Deep sighing breaths suggest acidosis whereas rapid shallow breathing suggests fluid overload and cardiac failure. Hiccoughs should be noted as |
| *Hiccoughs* | they are a sign of advanced renal failure. |
| *Fasciculation* | Irritability, fasciculation, tremor and fits are associated with advanced uraemia. |
| *Scratch marks* | Pruritus may be a major problem in patients with chronic renal failure, and scratch marks may be detected on the neck and trunk as well as the limbs. |
| *Bruising* | Easy bruising also occurs due to platelet dysfunction in renal failure. |
| *Rash* | The presence of a skin rash might suggest drug hypersensitivity as a cause of renal failure. |

### Face/Neck

| | |
|---|---|
| *Periorbital oedema* | Fluids tends to collect under the influence of gravity in tissue planes of low resistance, e.g. |

| | |
|---|---|
| *Uraemic frost (rare)* | around the eyes during the night and ankles during the day. Crystallisation of urea in the sweat — seen on the forehead as a 'frost' — may occur in the terminal stages of renal failure. |
| *Complexion* *Anaemia* | The muddy complexion of uraemic patients should be noted if present and anaemia and jaundice looked for in the conjunctiva and sclera. |
| *Jaundice* | Conditions that cause jaundice and uraemia include Weil's disease, Gram-negative septicaemia, drug toxicity and hypersensitivity, hepatorenal syndrome (associated with chronic liver disease) haemolytic-uraemic syndrome and incompatible blood transfusion. |
| *Jugular venous* *pressure* | The jugular venous pressure should be assessed during inspection of the neck. This will be elevated in fluid overload and might indicate chronic heart failure or its treatment as possible causes of renal failure. |
| *Tophi* | The ears should be inspected for gouty tophi and calcium deposits. |
| *Fundi* | The ocular fundi should be examined particularly for evidence of hypertension or diabetes mellitus. |
| **Hands** | Evidence of arthritis should be looked for and if present should raise the possibility of analgesic abuse. |
| *Skin turgor* | Skin turgor should be assessed by pinching the skin; this is diminished when there is a pre-renal component to the renal failure. |
| *Nails* *Brown arc* | The nails should be inspected for the distal brown arc of chronic renal failure (Lindsays's nails). |
| *Periungual infarcts* | A vasculitis such as those associated with systemic lupus erythematosus, rheumatoid arthritis or polyarteritis nodosa may be manifest by periungual infarcts. |
| *Nail-patella* *syndrome (rare)* | Split, deformed nails, with rudimentary patellae and iliac horns, make up the nail-patellae syndrome, which is inherited as an autosomal dominant trait and associated with chronic glomerulonephritis which may lead to renal failure. |
| *Calcium deposits* | Calcium deposits under the skin may be detected in patients with long-standing renal failure on dialysis. |
| *Fistulae* | A Cimino arterio-venous fistula may have been created as a means of vascular access in |

patients on haemodialysis. A thrill should be present over a patent fistula.

**Abdomen**
In patients being treated by continuous ambulatory peritoneal dialysis, a peritoneal cannula will be visible penetrating the abdominal wall connected to tubing and a bag. Except during 'exchange', the peritoneum will contain approximately 2 litres of dialysis fluid and appear swollen.

*Scars*
Scars of previous surgical operations should be noted as recent operations may be causally related to acute renal failure; previous renal transplants are another cause.

*Legs*
Oedema of the legs may be noted and severe generalised oedema may occur in the nephrotic syndrome.

**PALPATION**
The abdomen should be carefully palpated for the following:

**Kidneys**
The presence of two enlarged kidneys should suggest polycystic kidneys, amyloidosis or bilateral hydronephrosis. Enlargement of only one kidney should suggest absence of the other with vicarial hypertrophy, hypernephroma or unilateral hydronephrosis. More commonly in renal failure, small kidneys are found due to chronic glomerulonephritis, pyelonephritis, or hypertension. The fact that the kidneys are impalpable does not imply they are small. Renal angle tenderness should be looked for and suggests inflammation. A transplanted kidney is usually easily palpable in one or other iliac fossa.

**Bladder**
A palpable bladder in a patient with renal failure implies obstruction which is most commonly prostatic in origin (in men).

**Liver**
Patients with chronic liver disease may develop the hepatorenal syndrome. Hepatomegaly may also be found in Weil's disease, and diabetes mellitus (fatty liver) and polycystic disease.

**Spleen**
Although splenomegaly may rarely be found in patients with renal failure, it is important to be

| | able to differentiate the spleen from the left kidney (especially in clinical examinations). |
| *Tenderness* | In any patient undergoing peritoneal dialysis, abdominal tenderness is an important sign and may indicate peritonitis. Confirmation is made by identifying a cloudy dialysis effluent and by bacteriological culture. |

## General

| *Rectal examination* | A rectal examination should be performed, looking for benign prostatic hypertrophy or carcinoma of prostate or rectum. |
| *Fistula thrill* | The patency of a Cimino arteriovenous fistula should be confirmed by detecting an overlying thrill. |
| *Neuropathy* | In long-standing renal failure (without dialysis), a peripheral neuropathy may occur and should be sought. |

| **PERCUSSION** | Percussion has only limited application in these patients, but should be used to confirm a pleural effusion and peritoneal fluid if these are suspected. |

## AUSCULTATION

| *Heart murmurs* | Heart murmurs should be listened for, in particular 'flow' murmurs in anaemic patients. |
| *Pericardial rub* | A pericardial friction sound may be due to uraemic pericarditis or indicate an underlying connective tissue disorder (e.g. systemic lupus erythematosus). |
| *Bruit* | Patent arteriovenous fistulae should have an overlying bruit. A bruit may be heard over renal artery stenosis. |
| *Chest bases* | The presence of basal crepitations in the chest is a common manifestation of fluid overload in uraemic patients. |
| *Blood pressure* | Recording the blood pressure is an essential part of the examination and hypertension, if noted, may be primary (causal) or secondary in patients with renal failure. Postural hypotension may also occur, especially following dialysis. |

**Urine**

The examination of a patient with renal disease is incomplete without examining the urine. A fresh (warm) sample should be tested using
*Protein*
*Blood/glucose/pH*
'labstix' (or equivalent) for protein, blood, sugar and pH. Further biochemical analyses may be indicated in selected cases.
*Specific gravity*
The specific gravity should also be measured. The sample should then be inspected with the
*Colour*
naked eye and the colour and clarity noted. Cloudy urine is usually infected but may be due to phosphate or oxalate crystals in alkaline urine or urate crystals in acidic urine. Crystal clear urine is unlikely to be infected. Dark urine is usually either concentrated or contains blood or haemoglobin. 'Pseudohaematuria' may be due to drugs (e.g. rifampicin), dyes, beetroot, myoglobin, porphyrins and bilirubin. The urine should then be centrifuged, and the deposit inspected before the majority of the supernatant is discarded. The 'pellet' is then resuspended in the remaining urine and a drop of this 'concentrate' examined under a cover-glass microscopically, looking particularly for white and
*Cells*
red blood cells and casts. A few hyaline casts
*Casts*
should not be regarded as abnormal.
*Microorganisms*
Microorganisms may be identified in unstained preparations but the presence of pus cells is a more reliable indicator of urinary tract infection. If infection is suspected, bacteriological culture is essential to identify the microorganism and its antibiotic sensitivity.

# 15. DIABETES MELLITUS

Diabetic patients are prone to numerous complications and a complete medical examination is necessary for a full assessment to be made. The following approach should detect most problems. The emphasis is on detecting complications of the disease and its treatment.

## INSPECTION

### General

Hydration | The state of hydration should be noted and whether the patient is obese or has obviously lost weight.

Conscious level | The conscious level should be recorded and if the patient is confused or agitated consider hypoglycaemia, especially if associated with

Sweating | sweating and pallor.

Respiration | If the patient is breathing rapidly, or has 'air hunger' (deep, sighing inspiration and expiration), underlying acidosis should be suspected.

### Eyes

Visual acuity | Visual acuity should be checked.

Ocular movements | Check the external ocular movements. Mononeuritis and stroke are commoner among diabetics.

Iritis rubeosa | Iritis rubeosa, new vessel formation on the iris, may lead to glaucoma.

Cataracts | Cataracts occur at a younger age in diabetic patients. The snowflake-like deposits throughout the lens cortex that used to occur in adolescent diabetics are now rare. Examination of the fundi

Fundi | is essential and should always be carried out through dilated pupils. It is usually done at the end of the examination and the revelant abnormalities are listed in Table 3.2. Remember the different types of retinopathy that occur.

## Mouth

| | |
|---|---|
| *Candidiasis* | The presence of candidiasis should be noted as well as the state of dental hygiene. |

## Skin

| | |
|---|---|
| *Folliculitis* | Inspecting the skin may reveal folliculitis and |
| *Intertrigo* | other infections such as intertrigo. |
| *Moniliasis* | Moniliasis, particularly in the groin, may be noted as may fungal infections of the feet. |
| *Lipodystrophy* | Lipodystrophy — painless fat atrophy at sites of insulin injection — may be noted, particularly if older types of insulin preparations have been used. |
| *Insulin sensitivity* | Insulin sensitivity may manifest itself as tender lumps at injection sites. |
| *Necrobiosis lipoidica* | On the legs, necrobiosis lipoidica diabeticorum may be seen and is characterised by atrophy of subcutaneous collagen over the shins. The lesions are violet rings with a yellow periphery and scarring and atrophy at the centre. |
| *Brown spots* | Brown spots may also appear on the shins. |
| *Feet* | The feet should be examined for evidence of impaired circulation which tends to affect the toes first. |
| *Charcot's joints* | Denervation may give rise to Charcot's joints. |
| *Ulceration* | Ulceration in particular must be looked for and may be due to ischaemia and/or neuropathy. |

## PALPATION

| | |
|---|---|
| *Tachycardia* | The radial pulse should be palpated. A tachycardia may reveal an underlying infection or hypoglycaemia. |
| *Valsalva* | Lack of beat-to-beat pulse variation during a Valsalva manoeuvre may indicate autonomic neuropathy. |
| *Peripheral pulses* | All peripheral pulses should be carefully examined and may be absent in patients with severe atherosclerosis. |
| *Skin temperature* | Skin temperature of the feet should also be noted. |

| | |
|---|---|
| *Hepatomegaly* | Hepatomegaly may be present in diabetic patients due to fatty infiltration. |
| *Sensation* | Light touch and pinprick sensation should be assessed and are absent in peripheral neuropathy which is usually bilateral. |
| *Vibration*<br>*Proprioception* | Vibration sense and proprioception at the ankle may also be lost in peripheral neuropathy. Loss of sensation can be associated with ulceration over pressure points, even when pulses are present. |
| *Ankle jerk* | The ankle jerk is often absent when neuropathy is present. |
| *Mononeuritis* | A mononeuritis affecting most commonly the lateral popliteal, ulnar and oculomotor nerves may occur. |
| *Amyotrophy* | Weakness with wasting of the quadriceps, which may be asymetrical and painful, occurs in diabetic amyotrophy. |
| *Atonic bladder* | An enlarged atonic bladder might be detected in the abdomen. |

## PERCUSSION

Percussion has no particular place in the examination of diabetic patients except to confirm abnormalities such as pneumonia, pleural effusions and hepatomegaly where appropriate during the examination.

## AUSCULTATION

| | |
|---|---|
| *Vascular bruit* | Auscultation over the carotid, femoral and popliteal arteries for bruit should be performed, especially in patients with evidence of vascular disease. Remember that absence of bruit does not preclude the presence of atheromatous plaques. |
| *Heart*<br>*Chest* | Both the heart and lung fields should be auscultated for evidence of cardiac failure. Pneumonia occurs more often in diabetic patients and should be sought. |
| *Blood pressure* | The blood pressure should be recorded and any postural fall in pressure which occurs in autonomic neuropathy noted. Hypertension, if present, should be detected and treated accordingly. |

*Urinalysis*    Examination of the urine for ketones, glucose
and protein is an essential part of the
examination of diabetic patients. Urine and blood
glucose charts and records of $HbA_{1c}$ should also
be studied, if available.

# 16. THYROTOXICOSIS

Thyrotoxicosis in many cases is obvious at first glance but in others, especially the elderly, it may be manifest only by such changes as atrial fibrillation. Although the clinical diagnosis may appear obvious, it is essential to confirm it biochemically before starting anti-thyroid drug therapy. Examination of a hyperthyroid patient should be directed to confirming the diagnosis with positive typical findings and elucidating the cause.

## INSPECTION

### General

| | |
|---|---|
| *Hyperkinesia* | Thyrotoxic patients may be hyperkinetic and constant fidgeting may be noted. |
| *Stare* | There is often a characteristic staring appearance with sharp features. |
| *Weight loss* | Loss of weight may be apparent as may |
| *Sweating* | excessive sweating. |
| *Vitiligo* | Vitiligo is seen in thyrotoxicosis as well as other organ-specific autoimmune diseases. |
| *Mental state* | The patient may talk rapidly whilst their mental state may be normal, hypomanic or psychotic. |

### Eyes

| | |
|---|---|
| *Proptosis* | Proptosis should be looked for (see Ch. 3) and may be bilateral or unilateral. |
| *Exophthalmos* | Exophthalmos is recognised by a visible rim of sclera above and below the iris. |
| *Chemosis* | Chemosis (conjunctival oedema) and corneal |
| *Corneal scarring* | scarring may be noted if there is difficulty in completely closing the eyes. |

| | |
|---|---|
| *Lid retraction* | Lid retraction is noted when a rim of sclera is visible above the iris. |
| *Lid lag* | Lid lag should also be looked for (see Ch. 3). |
| *Globe lag* | Globe lag may also be detected when the upper eyelid moves up in advance of the eye on looking up. |
| *Ophthalmoplegia* | Ophthalmoplegia, with defective movement of one or more extrinsic eye muscles, should be looked for by testing eye movements. Failure of convergence is known as Moebius' sign. |

## Hands

| | |
|---|---|
| *Sweaty palms* | The palms are often hot and sweaty in thyrotoxicosis but cold and sweaty in simple anxiety. Palmar erythema may be present. |
| *Palmar erythema* | |
| *Tremor* | A fine tremor of the outstretched hands may be noted and a sheet of paper placed over the outstretched hand emphasises this. The tremor should be differentiated from that due to parkinsonism, alcoholism, and familial, benign essential tremors (see Ch. 1). |
| *Onycholysis* | The nails may exhibit onycholysis (elevation of the nail from the nail bed), and finger clubbing (thyroid achropachy) should be sought. |
| *Clubbing* | |

## Legs

| | |
|---|---|
| *Pretibial myxoedema* | Pretibial myxoedema is sometimes seen as raised, mauve-coloured patches over the shins and is invariably associated with eye signs and often with finger clubbing. It can occur in Graves' disease even when the patient is euthyroid. |

## PALPATION

### Pulse

| | |
|---|---|
| *Dysrhythmias* | Cardiac dysrhythmias may occur and in older people this may be the main presenting feature. Such dysrhythmias include sinus tachycardia, supraventricular tachycardia, atrial flutter, atrial fibrillation and ventricular ectopic beats. |

### Neck

| | |
|---|---|
| *Goitre* | A goitre may be present and its shape and size may help in the diagnosis (see Ch. 5). If large and |

| | |
|---|---|
| *Nodule* | smooth, Graves' disease is likely, whilst a hot nodule may appear as a solitary area of swelling or be part of a multinodular gland. Thyroid carcinoma does not usually cause thyrotoxicosis. |
| *Tenderness* | Tenderness over the thyroid indicates inflammation and viral thyroiditis may be associated with transient thyrotoxicosis. |
| *Trachea* | The position of the trachea should be checked to be sure it is central and retrosternal extension of the thyroid should be detected by palpation in the suprasternal notch. |

## Chest/Abdomen

| | |
|---|---|
| *Gynaecomastia*<br>*Hepatosplenomegaly* | Rarely, thyrotoxicosis is associated with gynaecomastia and hepatosplenomegaly. |
| **Muscles** | A proximal myopathy, tested by assessing the ease with which the patient rises from a chair, may be associated with thyrotoxicosis as may periodic paralysis and myasthenia gravis. |

## PERCUSSION

| | |
|---|---|
| *Retrosternal thyroid* | The upper aspect of the sternum should be percussed to detect dullness due to extension of thyroid tissue retrosternally. |

## AUSCULTATION

| | |
|---|---|
| *Bruit* | A bruit over the goitre is an important sign and adds considerable weight to the clinical diagnosis of thyrotoxicosis. |
| *Cardiac* | Auscultation of the heart will confirm a tachycardia and may reveal a gallop rhythm of incipient heart failure, a loud first heart sound and/or a systolic apical flow murmur associated with a hyperdynamic circulation. |
| *Wheezing/stridor* | Wheezing and inspiratory stridor may be produced by tracheal compression and should be listened for. |
| **Blood tests** | The full examination of patients with suspected thyrotoxicosis must include analysis of the blood for TSH, thyroxine and/or tri-iodothyronine levels. |

# 17. HYPERTENSION

The examination of patients with hypertension should include an attempt to identify any underlying causes, although it should be remembered that the cause of the commonest form — essential hypertension — is unknown. Sequelae of the disease and its treatment should also be sought.

## INSPECTION

Some causes of hypertension are suggested by typical appearances.

### Causes of Hypertension

*Cushing's syndrome*

Patients with Cushing's syndrome have a moon face, facial plethora, hirsutism, truncal obesity with wasted limbs, striae, bruising and gonadal atrophy. Children with this syndrome also may have short stature. Long-term treatment with corticosteroids has a similar effect.

*Acromegaly*

Acromegalic subjects frequently have coarse features with prognathia, a large tongue, large, spade-like hands and feet. Other features which may be apparent include sweating, bitemporal hemianopia and organomegaly.

*Coarctation of aorta (rare)*

Coarctation of the aorta may be associated with a recognisable syndrome such as Turner's or Marfan's syndrome. Look for active carotid and subclavian arterial pulsation and dilated pulsating vessels in the periscapular area.

*Phaeochromocytoma (rare)*

Phaeochromocytoma may occur in isolation or be associated with neurofibromatosis, parathyroid adenoma or medullary carcinoma of the thyroid (multiple endocrine adenomatosis type II) and von Hippel–Lindau syndrome. Signs that may indicate such associated conditions include multiple neurofibromata, café au lait spots, axillary freckles, mucosal neurofibromata (especially on the lips), Marfanoid habitus (in multiple endocrine adenomatosis IIB), and a goitre.

*Chronic renal failure*  Hypertension in chronic renal failure may be primary and causally related to the renal disease or secondary. Cutaneous manifestations include a 'muddy' complexion, purpura, scratch marks, uraemic frost and vascular access sites for haemodialysis.

## Effects of Hypertension

*Fundi*  The fundi should be examined for changes seen in hypertension. The classical subdivisions are as follows:

Grade I – arterial narrowing, increased light reflex of retina.

Grade II – vessel irregularity, arterio-venous nipping.

Grade III – soft, exudates, haemorrhages (usually flame shaped).

Grade IV – the above, plus papilloedema.

However, the classification into **mild** (Grades I and II) or **accelerated** (Grades III and IV) is clinically more useful.

*Cardiac failure*  The cardiovascular system must be examined for cardiac failure, looking for tachycardia, tachypnoea, an elevated JVP and ankle oedema (see Ch. 6).

*Hemiparesis*  Complications of hypertension such as hemiparesis may be easily recognisable.

## PALPATION

### Peripheral Pulses

*Large volume*  A large volume pulse may be associated with systolic hypertension and also occurs in 'high output' states (see Ch. 6).

*Radial-femoral delay*  In coarctation of the aorta, small and/or delayed femoral pulses may be present and periscapular vessels may also be palpable. Absent or reduced femoral pulses may also be found in aortic dissection.

## Praecordial Palpation

| | |
|---|---|
| *Apex beat* *Left ventricular heave* | Praecordial palpation may reveal a forceful apex beat with or without the left ventricular heave of left ventricular hypertrophy associated with long-standing hypertension. The apex beat may be displaced laterally and/or inferiorly in left ventricular dilatation. |
| *Double apical impulse* | A palpable fourth heart sound may also be detected as a double apical impulse in this situation. |
| *Right ventricular heave* | Pulmonary hypertension leads to right ventricular hypertrophy which produces a 'right ventricular heave' which is felt to the left of the sternum. |
| *Sacral/ankle oedema* | Pitting oedema should be looked for over the anterior aspect of the tibia and over the sacrum when cardiac failure is present as a complication of hypertension. |
| *Periorbital oedema* | Periorbital puffiness occurs, particularly in children, in glomerulonephritis, an uncommon cause of hypertension. |

## Abdomen

| | |
|---|---|
| *Kidneys* | The abdomen should be examined and the kidneys palpated. Bilateral renal enlargement is found in polycystic kidney disease while unilateral enlargement (the contralateral kidney) occurs in renal artery stenosis. Most other renal conditions associated with hypertension tend to produce small shrunken kidneys (which cannot be palpated). |
| *Adrenal tumours (rare)* | Adrenal tumours resulting in hypertension (phaeochromocytoma or adrenal adenoma) are rarely palpable. |

## AUSCULTATION

| | |
|---|---|
| **Blood Pressure** | The blood pressure must be measured (rather than relying on TPR charts at the foot of the bed), and record the arm used and the patient's position (erect, supine or sitting). In obese |

subjects, a large sphygmomanometer cuff must be used to avoid spuriously high readings. Most people recommend the use of phase 5 (disappearance of Korotkoff sounds) to represent diastolic blood pressure. Checking the systolic pressure by palpation over the radial artery should prevent the mistake of starting to record the systolic pressure in the auscultatory gap, an area of auscultatory silence below the systolic pressure, which exists in the occasional patient. Postural hypotension in a hypertensive patient should raise the possibility of an underlying phaeochromocytoma although more often it is related to drug therapy.

**Cardiac Murmurs**

Cardiac auscultation may reveal murmurs related to hypertension. Aortic regurgitation is associated with a large pulse pressure and systolic hypertension and is characterised by a blowing early diastolic murmur. Aortic or pulmonary flow murmurs may be heard in hyperdynamic states. A harsh continuous murmur radiating to the back between the scapulae with or without an aortic ejection click (bicuspid valve) may be audible in coarctation of the aorta.

*Basal crepitations*

Basal pulmonary crepitations in left ventricular failure are usually late inspiratory and medium pitched, and fail to clear after the patient is asked to cough. Radiological changes precede these clinical signs.

*Renal bruit*

Abdominal bruits are fairly common in the young and are usually innocent. The murmur of renal artery stenosis may be heard in the loins, both lateral regions and the midline. Bruits may also originate from aortic aneurysms which are associated with hypertension. Abdominal bruits, however, most commonly arise from an atheromatous aorta in patients who have neither renal artery stenosis nor an aortic aneurysm.

**Effects of Therapy**

Effects of therapy should be looked for and include gout, dehydration or muscle weakness (hypokalaemia) from diuretics; bradycardia, cardiac failure or cold peripheries from beta blockers; reflex tachycardia or flushing from vasodilators; postural hypotension from methyldopa, prazosin and others; cough from captopril; hypertrichosis from minoxidil; lupus erythematosus from hydralazine.

# 18. STROKE

When examining a patient who has suffered a stroke, while it is impossible to determine whether a cerebral infarct or haemorrhage is the cause, the likely location of the lesion causing the deficit must be determined. From the deficits detected it should be possible to predict the degree of disability. From the history of the onset of the acute stroke it should be possible to determine the likely prognosis in terms of survival and degree of recovery. In addition to the deficits the stroke has caused, examination should be aimed at detecting possible causes and risk factors, especially in young patients, and other disabling conditions which may compromise recovery.

## INSPECTION

| | |
|---|---|
| *Age* | The age of the patient should be noted — strokes are commonest in the elderly. |
| *Obesity* | Obesity is an obvious risk factor to note. |
| *Motor deficit* | The degree of deficit may be apparent, from a mild weakness (hemiparesis) barely detectable unless the patient is stressed or tired, to a dense paralysis (hemiplegia). The characteristic features associated with right and left hemipareses are shown in Table 18.1. |
| *Eye deviation* | Deviation of the eyes to the side of the weakness may occur. |
| *Level of consciousness* | This must be assessed, particularly in the acute stages, as impaired consciousness has a bad prognosis. |
| *Gait* | If the patient is conscious and can walk, much can be ascertained from observing the gait. Ask the patient to stand with feet together with the eyes |

**Table 18.1** Clinical features of different strokes

**Common features of strokes**
Cortical sensory loss
Face + arm > leg (middle cerebral art)
Leg worst (anterior cerebral art)
Face = arm = leg (internal capsule)
Eye deviation
Visual field defect
Dystonic postures (internal capsule)
Dense sensory loss (thalamic)
Crossed hemiplegia (brain stem)
Cerebellar signs, nystagmus, left ear hearing loss
(brain stem)
Dysarthria
Dysphagia

| **Right hemiplegia** | **Left hemiplegia** |
|---|---|
| Motor deficit | Motor deficit |
| Aphasia | Sensory inattention |
| | Denial, unconcern |
| | Constructional apraxia |
| | Dressing apraxia |
| | Spatial disorientation |
| | Impersistence |
| | Confusion |

| | |
|---|---|
| Ataxia | first open, then shut. If joint position sense is defective then loss of visual compensation by eye closure aggravates the sway; if the cerebellum is affected, closing the eyes will not alter the sway. |
| Turning | Turning may be affected. Parkinsonism can also be detected. |
| Posture | The dominant spasticity in the recovering stroke may give a characteristic posture with flexed, pronated arm and extended leg with foot drop. The face may be visibly affected. |
| Hypertension | Features of hypertension should be sought, since this is a major risk factor (see Ch. 17). |
| Facial appearance | Facial appearance may show clues such as malar flush in mitral stenosis, spider naevi and paper money telangiectasis in alcohol abuse (see Chs. 8 and 13). Drug addicts may be dishevelled and malnourished and may have injection marks. |
| Injection sites | |
| Deep venous thrombosis | Presence of DVT may be noted — it complicates the recovery phase and may also indicate a hypercoagulable state (e.g. antithrombin III deficiency, protein C deficiency, sickle-cell anaemia, familial plasminogen deficiency, lupus anticoagulant). |

**PALPATION**

Motor function is usually assessed in terms of power, tone, coordination and reflexes. The cranial nerves have already been dealt with (see Chs 3 and 4). Sensation is usually examined after power.

**Arms**
*Power*

Ask the patient to raise the arms to shoulder height or above the head. Weakness may prevent the movement or if the arms are held outstretched with the palms face up (with eyes closed) the pronator sign may be seen even before the arm starts to drift downward due to fatigue; the arm will gradually pronate and sometimes flex at the elbow due to the slight increase in tone of pronator muscles compared to supinator muscles.

In recovery from stroke the arm often takes longer to recover than the leg and may recover to a lesser degree.

Power should be recorded using a recognised scale, such as the MRC scale (Table 18.2). The different muscle groups can be tested in turn though this can be quite time-consuming.

In the hand the ability to perform various jobs such as lifting a cup then letting go, or fastening buttons, may be more revealing than detailed examinations of individual muscles.

*Crossed hemiplegia*

A classic feature of brain stem lesions is crossed hemiplegia where cranial nerve palsies on the contralateral side are produced at the level of the lesion.

*Tone*

With recovery the arm tends to have more tone in the flexor than the extensor muscles so particular attention should be paid to examining these. As recovery from the acute stroke occurs

Table 18.2  MRC scale for power assessment

| Degree of power | Scale |
| --- | --- |
| Normal | 5/5 |
| Mild weakness | 4/5 |
| Obvious weakness | 3/5 |
| Movement but not against gravity | 2/5 |
| Visible muscle contraction only | 1/5 |
| Paralysis | 0/5 |

a certain degree of spasticity may ensue. This can be demonstrated by 'clasp-knife' rigidity — often at the elbow. In a small minority of patients hypotonia continues throughout the recovery phase and they have a poor outlook in terms of functional recovery and may be at particular risk of developing subluxation of the shoulder joint.

*Reflexes*
*Hoffman's sign*
Deep tendon reflexes (biceps, supinator and triceps) should be tested. Hoffman's sign may occur (thumb flexes when distal middle finger is extended).

*Coordination*
Weakness of the arm may falsely suggest incoordination (in e.g. finger–nose test).

*Sensation*
This can be tested for by light touch, pin-prick and temperature sensation. A dense sensory

*Thalamic lesion*
loss is seen with thalamic lesions and with hemiplegia in adjacent internal capsule involvement.

*Spatial summation*
Sometimes a critical area of skin has to be stimulated to be perceived.

*Temporal summation*
Perception may occur only after a certain number of stimuli.

*Cortical sensory loss*
Test position sense, two-point localisation, graphasthesia (write different numbers on the palm) and stereognosis (use pen, key, coin).

*Sensory inattention*
This complicates non-dominant hemisphere lesions (usually left hemiparesis). The patient may neglect the left side of his body and his surroundings — the room, a picture. Check for extinction by double simultaneous sensory stimulation (with the patient's eyes closed touch both hands at once and ask which was touched); visual sensory extinction can be tested for in a similar way, when examining visual fields (see Ch. 3) by presenting fingers in each visual field at once. 'Thumb finding' is a useful test: with the patient's eyes shut take the right hand away and ask the patient to find the left thumb; the further away from the thumb the hand is the worse the degree of neglect.

*Constructional apraxia*
This also complicates non-dominant hemisphere lesions. Drawing a clock or copying a diagram will show this.

*Dressing apraxia*
Dressing apraxia may also be evident.

## Communication

*Spatial disorientation*  Spatial disorientation is a complication in non-dominant hemisphere lesions. Ask for local travel directions or analyse a picture.

*Speech Dysphagia*  Differentiate dysarthria from dysphasia and look for the presence of dysphagia.

*Aphasia*  Differentiate the types of aphasia (Table 18.3) by listening to speech output (fluent or not), reading and writing, ability to repeat, comprehend and name objects.

*Agnosia*  Disorders of recognition. Gerstmann's syndrome (left posterior parietal disease) includes agraphia, left–right confusion, finger agnosia, acalculia. There are a number of 'disconnection syndromes' with different combinations of deficits.

## Legs

*Power*  The predominant recovery pattern is with increased extensor tone. There may be foot drop (look for an ankle–foot orthosis). Flexion of the hip and knee and dorsiflexion of the foot may be the most revealing to test as they are less likely to recover fully than some other movements. Again power should be graded against gravity and/or resistance (Table 18.2). Examination of the patient flat on his or her back may cause a surprising degree of spasticity and may not reveal the patient's full potential.

*Tone*  Classically there is spasticity demonstrated by clasp-knife rigidity at the knee. Rotating the leg to and fro may show that the foot moves rigidly with the leg rather than with the passive inversion of the foot which occurs normally. In the rare patient with no occurrence of the normal spastic recovery pattern, the resultant flaccidity prevents a good functional outcome.

*Coordination*  The heel–shin test should be performed, though weakness of muscles can mimic incoordination.

*Reflexes*  These may be brisk; the deep tendon reflexes (knee and ankle) should be elicited and the plantar response (preferably using a fresh orange stick) recorded.

*Sensation*  This should be tested in a similar way to the upper limb.

**Table 18.3** Types of aphasia

| Type | Lesion | Characteristics |
|---|---|---|
| Broca's aphasia | Posterior third frontal gyrus (motor) | Speech slow, non-fluent, poor articulation<br>Phrase repetition poor<br>Aphasic writing<br>Object naming poor<br>Hemiparesis<br>Awareness, frustration, depression |
| Wernicke's aphasia | Posterior part of first temporal gyrus (close to auditory cortex) | Speech fluent, normal rhythm, articulation<br>Paraphasic errors, neologisms<br>Unable to comprehend written or verbal speech<br>Writing abnormal (cf. speech)<br>Object naming poor<br>Hemiparesis mild or absent<br>No realisation of deficit |
| Conduction aphasia | Arcuate fasciculus (temporal or parietal lesion) | Speech fluent<br>Information poorly conveyed<br>Paraphasic errors<br>Comprehension of simple sentences<br>Repetition affected<br>Difficulty naming objects<br>Written language impaired<br>Hemiparesis absent or mild |
| Anomic aphasia | Angular gyrus (encephalopathies, space occupying lesions) | Speech fluent<br>Paraphasic errors<br>Circumlocutions<br>Written language impaired<br>Difficulty naming objects<br>Understands written and spoken word<br>Comprehension and repetition normal<br>No hemiplegia |
| Global aphasia | Broca's and Wernicke's area (large middle cerebral artery infarcts) | Inability to comprehend or speak<br>Marked hemiparesis |

The speech cortex is usually on the left in right-handed people and in over 50% of left-handed people.

**Pulse**

Abnormalities of rate and rhythm must be detected. Acute arrhythmias may complicate an acute myocardial infarction (with resultant mural thrombus). Atrial fibrillation is a well-recognised risk factor for strokes.

**Neck**

*Carotid pulsations*

Presence or absence of carotid pulsation should be recorded.

**Praecordium**

*Thrills*

Palpable thrills may accompany murmurs (see below). Evidence of hypertension may be suggested by a forceful or displaced apex (see Ch. 6).

**PERCUSSION**

Percussion has little utility in the examination of a stroke patient except perhaps in detecting the complication of pneumonia.

**AUSCULTATION**

*Carotids*

Carotid bruits may be present but their absence does not exclude significant stenoses.

*Praecordium*
*Murmurs*

Mitral valve disease — classically mitral stenosis — is associated with strokes. Mitral valve prolapse should be excluded. Calcified and prosthetic valves, infective endocarditis, atrial myxoma, should be considered possible sources of thromboembolism. Cardiomyopathy and patent foramen ovale with paradoxical embolism are rare causes.

**FUNDOSCOPY**

*Cholesterol emboli*
*(rare)*
*Hypertensive*
*changes*

Cholesterol emboli are sometimes seen in retinal arteries on the same side as a diseased carotid artery, and in hypertensive patients the vascular changes may be less severe in the side with a stenosed carotid.

# 19. ATAXIA

Ataxia occurs when postural control is impaired leading to clumsy or uncoordinated movements. The two main causes are diseases of the cerebellum and of sensory nerves; brain stem, frontal lobe, spinal cord, peripheral nerve lesions should also be considered (Table 19.1).

## INSPECTION

*Gait ataxia*

Inspection of the patient's gait is essential and should be carried out first. Incoordination whilst walking is referred to as gait ataxia. Be careful to be standing nearby to catch the patient should he fall. As sensory ataxia can be mitigated to some extent by visual information, it is typically worse when the patient closes his eyes, whilst cerebellar ataxia is unchanged. Be careful not to misinterpret as ataxia the rather hesitant gait of elderly patients who suffer from drop attacks or vertigo. Patients with Parkinson's disease and other causes of parkinsonism may appear to have gait ataxia. Ataxia can occur in multiple strokes (état lacunaire) and in lesions of internal capsule or pons. More subtle incoordination in walking should be elicited by asking the patient to walk heel-to-toe, initially with eyes open and then closed.

*Romberg's sign*

Rombergism should then be assessed with the patient standing with feet together. Slight or even moderate swaying is not necessarily abnormal and a positive Romberg's sign should only be recorded if the patient sways so much with his eyes closed that he would fall without support or corrective measures. Rombergism is a sign of posterior column

**Table 19.1** Causes of ataxia

*CEREBELLUM*

Infarct, haemorrhage, tumour; alcohol, occult malignancy; spinocerebellar degeneration, acute cerebellitis.

*FRONTAL LOBE*

Tumour, anterior cerebral artery thrombosis, aneurysm of anterior communicating artery, hydrocephalus.

*SUBCORTICAL*

Multiple strokes, internal capsule or pons.

*BRAINSTEM*

Cerebrovascular accident, multiple sclerosis.

*SPINAL CORD*

Cervical spondylosis, multiple sclerosis, vitamin $B_{12}$ deficiency, syringomyelia, tumour, tabes dorsalis, amyotrophic lateral sclerosis.

*MUSCLE*

Myopathy: congenital (dystrophy), acquired (polymyositis, thyroid myopathy).

*CHRONIC PROGRESSIVE ATROPHY*

Friedreich's ataxia, Charcot-Marie-Tooth, Huntington's chorea, Refsum's syndrome, meningeal leukaemia.

*ACUTE FORM*

Alcohol, lead, post-ictal, sickle-cell crisis, SLE.

---

damage. Patients with cerebellar lesions tend to lean or fall towards the side of the lesion. Such a tendency can be displayed by asking the patient to walk in circles, which become increasingly small when turning towards the side of the lesion and increasingly large in the opposite direction. Patients with frontal ataxia tend to fall backwards. (Look for other signs of frontal lobe dysfunction — perseveration, grasp and suck reflexes, incontinence, slowness of thought.)

**Colour**

Vitiligo, pallor and lemon-yellow pigmentation may occur in pernicious anaemia, which, along with other causes of peripheral neuropathy, may cause sensory ataxia. Sickle-cell anaemia should be considered.

**Eyes**

*Pupils*
*Ptosis*

The eyes should be closely inspected for Argyll Robertson pupils and bilateral ptosis seen in tabes dorsalis.

| | |
|---|---|
| *Nystagmus* | Nystagmus is coarse and jerking (maximal to the side of the lesion) or rotatory in cerebellar disease while 'ataxic' nystagmus occurs in multiple sclerosis (see Ch.3). Conjunctival and |
| *Telangiectasia* | skin telangiectasia occurs in the rare inherited disorder, ataxia telangiectasia. |

**Head**

| | |
|---|---|
| *Position* | Tilting of the head may be present due to cerebellar hemisphere damage or to help compensate for astigmatism. |
| *Titubation* | Tremor or titubation of the head is seen in some patients with cerebellar disease. |
| *Alcoholism* | Alcoholic facies or cutaneous stigmata of alcoholic liver disease (see Ch. 13) should suggest alcohol as a cause of cerebellar disease, whilst finger clubbing may be related to a primary lung tumour with cerebellar metastases. |
| *Myxoedema* | Myxoedema may cause cerebellar degeneration and should be remembered when examining ataxic patients. |
| *Friedreich's ataxia* | Pes cavus, pes equinovarus and kyphoscoliosis should suggest Friedreich's ataxia, an autosomal recessively-inherited spinocerebellar disorder which may present in childhood or adolescence. |
| *Cerebellar degeneration* | Other degenerative conditions involving the cerebellum (e.g. spinocerebellar and olivo-pontocerebellar atrophy) occur in later life. |

**ACTIVE MOVEMENT**

| | |
|---|---|
| *Gait ataxia* | See above. |
| *Truncal ataxia* | A tendency to fall backwards whilst sitting or standing is typical of midline cerebellar lesions and referred to as truncal ataxia. |
| *Limb ataxia* | Coordination in the upper limbs should be checked systematically. First, observe the patient's fully outstretched hands looking for |
| *Hyperpronation* | hyperpronation and tremor of cerebellar disease |
| *Tremor* | and then apply and suddenly remove pressure to the outstretched arms. This leads to marked |
| *Over-correction* | over-correction of the initial position in patients with cerebellar disease. In Parkinson's disease a resting tremor may be abolished on exercise. |

The patient should then be asked to touch the tip of his nose with the index finger of both hands in turn with the eyes open initially and then closed.

*Intention tremor*    An intention tremor, a tremor of increasing amplitude as the hand reaches the target, is typical of cerebellar disease. A more subtle test of coordination involves asking the patient to touch first the tip of his nose and then the examiner's finger which is moved in various directions.

*Past pointing*    Overshooting the target or past pointing (dysmetria) is typical of cerebellar lesions. Coordination in the legs can be assessed by asking the patient to run the right foot slowly and accurately up the front of the left shin to the knee and vice versa.

## Rapid Simple Movements

*Dysdiadochokinesia*    Dysdiadochokinesia, the inability to perform rapid simple alternating movements, should be assessed. The most usual method of checking for this is to ask the patient to tap one hand as fast as possible on the back of the other and vice versa. The same test can be used for the feet, usually asking the patient to tap his foot rapidly against the examiner's hand. Rapid alternating pronation and supination at the wrist is a further test for dysdiadochokinesia. These tests tend to be performed better on the dominant side and this should always be checked. Unilateral incoordination or ataxia can easily be identified using these tests. Be careful not to over-interpret mild bilateral incoordination. The patient's writing should also be observed as it tends to become larger and more untidy in patients with cerebellar disease while micrographia is a feature of parkinsonism.

## Passive Movement

*Tone*    Tone should be assessed at the wrists, elbows, knees and ankles. Reduced tone, particularly if unilateral, is suggestive of ipsilateral cerebellar disease. Acute pyramidal lesions can also cause hypotonia and should be excluded. In parkinsonism there is increased tone (lead pipe) with cogwheeling if there is a tremor present.

## Reflexes

*Pendular*

The tendon reflexes should be elicited. In peripheral neuropathy they will be absent, whilst in cerebellar disease they tend to be slower and 'pendular'.

*Delayed relaxation*

Delayed relaxation of the reflexes occurs in hypothyroidism, which may be the cause of cerebellar ataxia.

*Plantar reflexes*

The plantar reflexes should be checked and may be dorsiflexor and associated with absent ankle jerks in subacute combined degeneration, diabetes mellitus, Friedreich's ataxia, taboparesis and motor neurone disease. All but the last may cause ataxia.

## Sensation

*Fine touch and proprioception*

Fine touch and proprioception should be checked to exclude a sensory neuropathy, causes of which include diabetes mellitus, pernicious anaemia, alcoholism and carcinomatous neuropathy.

## Speech

*Staccato*

The quality of the patient's speech should be assessed. In cerebellar disease, it tends to be 'staccato'. Rapid repetition of words such as 'cat' or 'tick-tock' may make this obvious.

*Scanning*

Mutiple sclerosis may cause 'scanning' speech due to combined cerebellar and pyramidal lesions.

The patient should be asked if he is epileptic and/or taking phenytoin, since this may cause ataxia with high blood levels.

## FURTHER EXAMINATION

*Fundoscopy*

Evidence of raised intracranial pressure due to a posterior fossa lesion should be sought at fundoscopy. Optic atrophy and retinal pigmentation may be due to Refsum's disease, an autosomal recessive disorder which may cause ataxia in association with deafness, muscular atrophy and peripheral neuropathy. If the results of the examination suggest that the ataxia may be related to a carcinoma, the primary should be sought, the commonest being a bronchial carcinoma.

# 20. CONFUSED PATIENT

It is essential to identify whether a patient is clinically confused; a screening procedure is required to do this. The Aberdeen MSQ (Table 20.1), the Clifton Assessment Scale, and the Mini Mental State examination are all quick tests. It is essential to differentiate acute confusion (delirium) from chronic confusion (dementia), as the former is more likely to have a treatable cause. Some forms of dementia are treatable, however, and these must be actively sought. In some patients with an underlying dementia, a delirium is also present.

Many clues as to the cause come from the history given by carers, e.g. getting lost, misuse of words, sloppy habits, ataxia, incontinence, toxin exposure, trauma, depression, etc.

## DEFINE THE MENTAL STATE

*State of consciousness*

The state of consciousness may be diminished in a metabolic disorder or with a space-occupying lesion.

Table 20.1  A simple screening test for confusion (Aberdeen MSQ)

| | |
|---|---|
| Today's date? | Age? |
| Today's month? | Month of birth? |
| Today's year? | Year of birth? |
| This town? | Present Prime Minister? |
| Present situation? | Previous Prime Minister? |

Total (out of 10) Normal = 7 or over

| | |
|---|---|
| *Delirium* | Delirium rather than dementia is suggested by inattention, sleep disturbances, fluctuating symptoms, perceptual abnormalities and increased autonomic activity. |
| *Screening test* | A screening test (see Table 20.1) |
| *Orientation* | should be used. Orientation in time, place and person should be noted. |
| *Aphasia* | Aphasia may present as a confusion; check speech and writing (see Ch. 18). |
| *Memory* | Recent memory is often more severely affected: place money under patient's pillow and test later, check knowledge of current events. Ask about historical events to check distant memory. |
| *Calculation* | Give a practical problem, e.g. if chocolate bars cost 26p, how many bars can you get for £1? |
| *Pictures* | Interpreting magazine pictures can be helpful. In visual agnosia, integration is a problem. Constructional apraxia may prevent copying of designs. |
| *Abstraction* | Give practical problems, e.g. similarity between orange and ball. |
| *Mood* | Sadness or dejection should be noted, suggesting depressed mood or depression (depression can cause pseudodementia and dementia can cause depression, especially where there is insight). Inappropriate mood elevation may suggest mania or thyrotoxicosis. Fearfulness and paranoia should be noted. |
| *Emotional lability* | Emotional lability may suggest cerebrovascular disease. |

## INSPECTION

| | |
|---|---|
| *Dress* | The state of dress may give a clue. Dementia may cause poor dress sense and clothes may not be cared for. Depression, too, tends to diminish dress sense. |
| *General* | Full examination is essential. Particular attention should be paid to evidence of diseases of the liver (see Chs 8 and 13), kidneys (see Ch. 14), respiratory system (see Ch. 7), heart (see Ch. 6), and thyroid (see Ch. 16). |

## PALPATION

| | |
|---|---|
| *Abdomen* | Evidence of hepatomegaly and renal enlargement |

|  | should be sought. Splenomegaly is very rare in pernicious anaemia. |
| Blood pressure | Hypotension might be seen in shock state (e.g. silent acute myocardial infarction, septicaemia). Hypertension is a risk factor for atherosclerosis; it is seen in multi-infarct dementia and atherosclerotic encephalopathy (Binswanger's syndrome). |
| Heart failure | Heart failure can also cause Binswanger's syndrome. |

## Central Nervous System

| Primitive reflexes | Primitive reflexes — suck, snout, rooting, grasp reflexes — may be present with frontal lobe damage (e.g. in Alzheimer's disease, tumours). |
| Sensory signs | Sensory signs might suggest pernicious anaemia, thiamine deficiency, syphilis or diabetes mellitus. |
| Drowsiness | Drowsiness might suggest a subdural haematoma or over-sedation (e.g. phenothiazines). Liver failure is also characterised by drowsiness. |
| Gait | Walking apraxia with ataxia, urinary incontinence and dementia suggests normal pressure hydrocephalus, though they are more commonly seen in Alzheimer's disease. Spasticity of the lower limbs can occur in normal pressure hydrocephalus but is commoner in multi-infarct dementia; Creutzfeldt–Jakob disease is a rarer cause. Parkinsonism is common in Alzheimer's disease, while dementia may occur in Parkinson's disease. The dementia of AIDS can have any combination of these signs. |
| Chorea | Choreiform movements may be seen in Huntington's chorea. |

## PERCUSSION

| Lungs | Percussion of the chest will help to define any respiratory disease (see Ch. 7) and should be used to confirm organomegaly, e.g. hepatomegaly. |

## AUSCULTATION

Particular attention should be paid to the respiratory and cardiovascular systems.

| | |
|---|---|
| *Chest* | Coarse crackles (or crepitations) may suggest pneumonia and this can be confirmed as previously described (see Ch. 7). Wheezes (rhonchi) might suggest an exacerbation of obstructive airways disease. |
| *Heart* | Cardiac murmurs (see Ch. 6) occur in infective endocarditis. Aortic sclerotic murmurs are common in generalised atherosclerosis. |
| *Carotid bruits* | Carotid bruits reflect atherosclerosis and might indicate cerebrovascular disease. Bruits may be |
| *Cranial bruits* | heard overlying intracranial vascular malformations. |

# 21. ARTHRITIS

Arthritis is a common disorder and arthritic patients are frequently used in clinical examinations. There are numerous causes of arthritis and more than one disease process may be present in an individual patient (e.g. septic monoarthritis in a patient with rheumatoid disease).

## INSPECTION

### Sex

The sex of the patient is important and influences the differential diagnosis of rheumatic diseases: Reiter's disease, gout and ankylosing spondylitis are much commoner in men whilst systemic lupus erythematosus, systemic sclerosis and rheumatoid arthritis are commoner in women.

### Face

*Cushingoid*
*Alopecia*
*Butterfly rash*
*Heliotrope rash*

*Malnourished*

*Gouty tophi*

Cushingoid facies may be related to steroid treatment, whilst alopecia and a 'butterfly rash' occur in systemic lupus erythematosus.
A heliotrope rash of the cheeks and forehead (and knuckles) occurs in dermatomyositis.
Malnourishment may mean underlying tuberculosis.
Gouty tophi should be looked for around the cartilage of the ear.

### Eyes

*Anaemia*
*Uveitis*

The eyes should be inspected for the conjunctival pallor of anaemia and uveitis in juvenile rheumatoid arthritis, ankylosing spondylitis, Behçet's and Reiter's syndromes.

| | |
|---|---|
| *Dry eyes* | Dry eyes occur with Sjögren's syndrome and occasionally scleromalacia in rheumatoid arthritis. |
| *Cataracts* | Cataracts may be due to steroid or chloroquine therapy. |

## Mouth

| | |
|---|---|
| *Systemic sclerosis* | Tightening of the skin around the mouth, frequently associated with telangiectasia, occurs in systemic sclerosis. |
| *Xerostomia* | Xerostomia (dry mouth) is seen in Sjögren's syndrome, while buccal ulceration is seen in Behçet's syndrome and inflammatory bowel disease. |

## Skin

| | |
|---|---|
| *Rashes* | Rashes should be looked for specifically and in good light as they are sometimes difficult to see, especially if fading. They frequently represent drug hypersensitivity but also occur in juvenile rheumatoid arthritis, rheumatic fever, secondary syphilis, brucellosis, and Henoch–Schönlein purpura. In gonococcal septicaemia, skin lesions on the periphery may be papular, pustular, haemorrhagic or necrotic. |
| *Psoriasis* | The skin eruption and nail pitting of psoriasis must not be missed (see Ch. 1). |
| *Erythema marginatum* | Erythema marginatum may occur in rheumatic fever. |
| *Erythema nodosum* | Erythema nodosum appearing as tender red nodules over the shins may accompany polyarteritis nodosa, rheumatoid arthritis, rheumatic fever, sarcoidosis, mycoplasmal infection and drug hypersensitivity, all of which may cause an arthritis. |
| *Livedo reticularis* | Livedo reticularis, a reticulate pattern of skin marking similar to erythema ab igne ('Granny's tartan') is associated with polyarteritis nodosa and systemic lupus erythematosus. |
| *Purpura* | Purpura may be seen in Henoch–Schönlein purpura and in thrombocytopenia, secondary to treatment (gold, penicillamine) in rheumatoid arthritis. |
| *Ecchymoses* | Ecchymoses may be seen with steroid therapy and in scurvy, and bleeding can affect large joints (hips and knees). Haemarthroses may occur in haemophilia but there are usually few external signs of bleeding. |

| | |
|---|---|
| *Scars* | Scars of previous orthopaedic surgery should be noted, as should multiple abnormal scars or enterostomies, suggestive of inflammatory bowel disease. |
| *Pigmentation (rare)* | Skin pigmentation may be seen in Whipple's disease, along with lymphadenopathy, pyrexia and a migratory polyarthritis. The latter is frequently the first symptom of the disorder. |

**Genitalia**

| | |
|---|---|
| *Ulceration* | Genital ulceration occurs in Behçet's syndrome, |
| *Urethral discharge* | while urethral discharge occurs in gonorrhoea |
| *Circinate balanitis* | and Reiter's syndrome where circinate balanitis also may be noted. |

**Joints**

All major joints should be inspected and compared with the opposite side looking for:
1. swelling
2. erythema
3. deformity
4. associated abnormalities such as bursitis, muscle wasting and rheumatoid nodules.

The hands, elbows and feet in particular must be carefully examined. The pattern of joint involvement in different diseases is outlined in Table 21.1. A single red, swollen painful joint in a patient with a chronic arthritis may signal infection of the joint.

**Hands** (see Ch. 1)

| | |
|---|---|
| *Clubbing* | Finger clubbing may occur in Whipple's disease and chronic inflammatory bowel disease, both of which may have joint manifestations, and in hypertrophic pulmonary osteoarthropathy associated with pulmonary suppuration and tumours. |
| *Nail fold infarcts* | Nail fold infarcts are seen in active rheumatoid arthritis and dermatomyositis. |
| *Raynaud's phenomenon* | Raynaud's phenomenon and sclerodactyly are features of systemic sclerosis, while subcutaneous calcified nodules in addition in the hands suggest CRST syndrome (calcinosis, Raynaud's, sclerodactyly, telangiectasia). |
| *Heberden's nodes* *Bouchard's nodes* | Exostoses such as Heberden's nodes (distal interphalangeal joints) and Bouchard's nodes (proximal interphalangeal joints) are seen in |

| | |
|---|---|
| *Gouty tophi* | osteoarthrosis, whilst gouty tophi are seen in the arthropathy of gout. In chronic gout there may be deformity. |
| *Arthritis mutilans* | Arthritis mutilans is a severe chronic form of psoriatic arthropathy. |
| *Ulnar deviation* | Rheumatoid arthritis tends to produce ulnar deviation of the fingers, and subluxation at the metacarpophalangeal joints is typical, as are |
| *Deformities* | 'swan-neck' and 'boutonnière' deformities of fingers, which are due to tendon damage. |
| *Muscle wasting* | Oedema of the hands and muscle wasting are also frequently seen in rheumatoid arthritis, which tends to cause spindle-shaped swollen fingers and spares the distal interphalangeal joints, unlike osteoarthrosis and psoriatic arthropathy (see Table 21.1). |
| *Tinel's sign* | Carpal tunnel syndrome may result in thenar wasting and produce a positive Tinel's sign (tingling if the median nerve at the wrist is tapped). |

## Elbows

| | |
|---|---|
| *Nodules* | Subcutaneous rheumatoid nodules are frequently found at the elbow and should be looked for specifically. The rheumatic nodule of acute rheumatic fever is characteristically found over the back of the skull. |
| *Bursitis* | Olecranon bursitis should be looked for (in rheumatoid arthritis, ankylosing spondylitis and gout), as well as deformity. |
| *Deformity* | |
| *Psoriasis* | Psoriatic plaques are frequently found on the elbow (i.e. the extensor surfaces). |

## Feet

| | |
|---|---|
| *Rheumatoid arthritis* | Characteristic deformity of the feet and toes is seen in rheumatoid arthritis with dorsal subluxation of the toes exposing the metatarsal heads to pressure during walking, which may lead to ulceration. Hallux valgus also typically develops. |
| *Gout* | The swollen, red, tender, painful great toe (prodagra) typical of an acute attack of gout should not be missed nor confused with an inflamed bunion. |
| *Keratoderma blenorrhagica* | The soles of the feet must be inspected for keratoderma blenorrhagica, the lesions of which appear initially as vesicles and later as sterile |

---

**Table 21.1** Typical joint distribution and associated features of various arthritides

*RHEUMATOID ARTHRITIS (RA)*

Hands (MCP & PIP), feet, wrists, knees, shoulders, ankles, hips, cervical spine, temperomandibular joint. Symmetrical polyarticular, nodules, muscle wasting.

*Assoc.* leg ulcers, scleritis, Sjögren's syndrome, vasculitis, valve and myocardial lesions, pleural effusions, alveolitis, lymphadenopathy, splenomegaly, carpal tunnel syndrome, neuropathy, anaemia, amyloid.

*JUVENILE RHEUMATOID ARTHRITIS*

Joints as RA — less symmetrical, sometimes monoarticular.

*Assoc.* lymphadenopathy, splenomegaly, pericarditis, rash, iritis, anaemia, growth retardation.

*OSTEOARTHROSIS*

Hands (DIP & PIP), thumb, spine, knees, hips. Symmetrical polyarticular

*Assoc.* Heberden's (DIP) and Bouchard's (PIP) joints (osteophytes).

*REITER'S SYNDROME*

Knees, ankles, feet (MTP), sacro-iliitis. Asymmetrical polyarticular

*Assoc.* urethritis, balanitis, keratoderma blenorrhagica, conjunctivitis, calcaneal spurs, plantar fasciitis.

*ANKYLOSING SPONDYLITIS*

Sacro-iliitis, spine, ribs, also hips, knees, ankles.

*Assoc.* uveitis, aortic incompetence, alveolitis.

*GOUT*

Great toe (MTP), hands (DIP, PIP), gouty tophi. Asymmetrical, oligoarticular. (Negatively birefringent needle-shaped urate crystals.)

*PSEUDOGOUT*

Knees, other large joints. Asymmetrical, oligoarticular. (Positively birefringent brick-shaped pyrophosphate crystals.) Idiopathic or in haemachromatosis, hyperparathyroidism, acromegaly.

*PSORIASIS*

Hands (DIP) especially, may simulate RA: sacroiliitis.

*Assoc.* nail pitting, psoriatic rash (elbows and knees).

*SYSTEMIC LUPUS ERYTHEMATOSUS*

Joints as RA (less deformity). Symmetrical, polyarticular.
*Assoc.* rash, renal failure, pericarditis, cardiac lesions, pleurisy, pulmonary fibrosis, neuropathy, fits, psychosis.

*SYSTEMIC SCLEROSIS*

Fingers especially, symmetrical.

*Assoc.* skin bound down, oedematous and smooth, telangiectasia, ulceration, renal failure, Raynaud's and Sjögren's syndromes.

---

MCP = metacarpophalangeal; PIP = proximal interphalangeal;
DIP = distal interphalangeal; MTP = metatarsophalangeal.

pustules with hyperkeratosis. If this is found the other features of Reiter's disease (conjunctivitis, uveitis, urethritis, circinate balanitis, mouth ulcers and Achilles' tendinitis) must be looked for.

*Ankle oedema*     Ankle oedema may be a feature of nephrotic syndrome related to gold and penicillamine therapy but may simply be due to immobility.

*Leg ulcers*       Leg ulcers may complicate the vasculitis of active rheumatoid arthritis.

## Posture

*Pelvic tilt*      Abnormalities of posture may be due to arthritic processes. Tilting of the pelvis may suggest underlying osteoarthrosis or rheumatoid arthritis of the hip. There will often be a compensatory scoliosis.

*Knee*             A genu valgum deformity may complicate a deforming knee arthropathy.

*Spine*            In ankylosing spondylitis a characteristic fixed stooped posture may be noted.

## PALPATION

*Joints*           After inspection, the joints should be palpated. Enquire of the patient whether any joint is tender before proceeding and handle with care—do not cause pain. There is not time, particularly during an examination, to palpate all joints and special attention should therefore be directed to deformed and swollen joints where particular care is required.

*Tenderness*       The degree of tenderness should be assessed as well as soft tissue swelling. Calcaneal tenderness is noted in Reiter's syndrome and ankylosing spondylitis.

*Nodules*          Rheumatoid nodules along the radius may be missed on inspection and should be sought specifically by palpation.

*Telescoping*      Telescoping of the fingers can be demonstrated in psoriatic arthritis mutilans, though this sign can be present in rheumatoid arthritis.

*Effusions*        Joint effusions may be identified clinically and should be looked for particularly in the knee. Conditions which may simulate a knee effusion are prepatellar bursitis and cellulitis.

*Patella tap*

Tests used to detect presence of fluid in the knee joint include the patella tap where the patella can be bounced off underlying bone once fluid in the suprapatellar pouch is diverted into the knee joint by manual compression. This test identifies moderate volumes. Smaller volumes can be identified by pressing over the hollow on one side of the patella and watching for filling of the opposite hollow. Large volumes are usually obvious, but can be confirmed by transmitting a fluid impulse from around the ligamentum patellae below the patella to the swelling above the patella.

*Hip*

In osteoarthrosis of the hip, there may be apparent shortening of the leg, and measuring the distance from the medial malleolus to the anterior superior iliac spine will help differentiate from true shortening. Thomas' test will reveal flexion deformity, i.e. flexion of the unaffected hip straightens the lumbar spine and leads to elevation of the affected leg.

## Movement

*Active/passive*

Joints should be put through their range of movements initially actively (by the patient) and then passively, and the degree of movement recorded.

*Hypermobility*

Hypermobility of joints should be looked for, particularly of the fingers and wrist, and occurs in Marfan's or Ehlers–Danlos syndrome, osteogenesis imperfecta, and homocystinuria. It may also be idiopathic or associated with deformity as in rheumatoid arthritis or Charcot's joints (grossly disordered painless joints seen in the knee and ankle in tabes dorsalis and diabetes mellitus and in the arm in syringomyelia).

*Crepitus*

Instability should be looked for during passive joint manipulation. Crepitus may be felt during movement of damaged joints.

Flexion, extension and rotation of the spine should be included if ankylosing spondylitis is not to be missed, and sacro-iliac joint tenderness (on springing the pelvis) may be seen early in ankylosing spondylitis and Reiter's syndrome.

**Abdomen**

*Splenomegaly*

The abdomen should be palpated in patients with evidence of rheumatoid disease, looking specifically for the splenomegaly of Felty's syndrome and juvenile rheumatoid arthritis.

*Kidneys*

Palpable kidneys may occur in amyloidosis associated with rheumatoid arthritis.

**PERCUSSION**

Percussion is of limited value in examining patients with joint disease, except in identifying areas of tenderness over the spine (percussing with the ulnar aspect of the clenched fist), and in detecting pleural effusions, which occur in systemic lupus erythematosus and rheumatoid disease.

**AUSCULTATION**

Creaking and clicking during movement of damaged joints is often audible without the stethoscope.

*Heart murmurs*

Cardiac auscultation may detect cardiac murmurs in acute rheumatic fever (Carey Coombs), ankylosing spondylitis and tertiary syphilis (aortic regurgitation). A pericardial rub may be heard in rheumatoid disease and systemic lupus erythematosus whilst pulmonary crepitations occur in ankylosing spondylitis (apical) and rheumatoid disease, systemic lupus erythematosus and sarcoidosis (basal).

*Pericardial rub*

*Crepitations*

# 22. HIV INFECTION

HIV infection has replaced syphilis as the great masquerader and should be included in the differential diagnosis of numerous conditions. The possibility of HIV infection should be considered in all patients, especially those with a history of intravenous drug abuse or homosexuality. Patients with unusual infections are also likely candidates though HIV patients generally have common infections. Confidence in examining the HIV patient is paramount and specific precautions are needed only when there is an open wound or body tissue is exposed. Patients with HIV infection may present at many stages short of full-blown AIDS and the whole clinical spectrum will be considered below. (See Table 22.1 for CDC Classification System for HIV Infections.)

## INSPECTION

**General**

A hypercatabolic wasting syndrome may be present even in the absence of secondary infectious disease. There is sometimes an appearance of premature ageing.

**Skin**

*Infections*

Minor opportunistic infections are common and include viral warts, molluscum contagiosum, folliculitis, impetigo and fungal infections. Severe

*Seborrhoeic dermatitis*

*Kaposi's sarcoma*

seborrhoeic dermatitis is also recognised. Purple nodules, frequently at different sites, are typical of Kaposi's sarcoma.

**Arms**

Marks over veins should be specifically looked

**Table 22.1**  CDC classification system of HIV infections

| | |
|---|---|
| Group I | **Acute infection**: associated with HIV seroconversion |
| Group II | **Asymptomatic infection**: must have had no previous signs or symptoms that would have led to classification in groups III or IV |
| Group III | **Persistent generalised lymphadenopathy** |
| Group IV | **Other disease** (subgroup classification independent of lymphadenopathy) |

Subgroups

A  **Constitutional disease**: fever > 1 month, weight loss > 10% base line, diarrhoea > 1 month

B  **Neurological disease**: dementia, myelopathy, peripheral neuropathy

C  **Secondary infectious diseases**
C1: those specified in CDC surveillance definition
C2: others (oral candida, oral hairy leukoplakia, multidermatomal herpes zoster, recurrent salmonella bacteraemia, tuberculosis)

D  **Secondary cancers**: Kaposi's sarcoma, non-Hodgkin's lymphoma, primary cerebral lymphoma

E  **Other conditions**: e.g. thrombocytopenia, lymphoid interstitial pneumonitis

---

| | |
|---|---|
| *Drug abuse* | for as evidence of intravenous drug abuse. |

## Mouth

| | |
|---|---|
| *Infections* | This should be closely inspected for thrush (candidiasis) which may also affect pharynx and oesophagus, impairing swallowing. Aphthous ulcers and gingivitis are also common. Mucocutaneous ulceration is characteristic of herpes simplex virus infection. |
| *Leukoplakia* | Oral hairy leukoplakia is not uncommon and classically affects the lateral border of the tongue. Kaposi's sarcoma should be specifically looked for in the mucous membranes and soft palate and squamous carcinoma around the lips. |

## Eyes

Chorioretinitis, if present, represents disseminated cytomegalovirus infection. A non-specific retinopathy with exudates may be present.

## Anogenital region

| | |
|---|---|
| *Ulcers* | Perianal ulceration due to herpes simplex virus infection may be present. |
| *Warts*<br>*Carcinoma* | Perianal warts and squamous carcinoma are recognised. |

| | |
|---|---|
| **PALPATION**<br>*Lymph nodes* | Generalised lymphadenopathy is common in HIV infection. Nodes larger than 1 cm in diameter, present in two or more extra inguinal sites for at least 3 months, are found in the persistent generalised lymphadenopathy syndrome. In many other patients lesser degrees of lymphadenopathy may exist. Specific examination should be made of the neck (especially post-cervical nodes), axillary as well as inguinal regions. The nodes are usually symmetrical, mobile and non-tender. Larger non-mobile nodes may suggest involvement by lymphoma, or Kaposi's sarcoma. |
| **Abdomen** | |
| *Hepatomegaly* | This should be carefully examined for hepatomegaly secondary to hepatitis due to mycobacteria, cytomegalovirus or drug induced. |
| *Splenomegaly* | Splenomegaly is not uncommon. Careful examination of the remainder of the abdomen should be undertaken to exclude intra-abdominal neoplasia. |
| **CNS** | Encephalopathy manifesting as dementia and myelopathy occurs in patients with AIDS. Cognition should be assessed (see Ch. 20) documenting the level of consciousness, orientation, attention and concentration (e.g. by serial subtraction of 7 from 100), memory (recall of recent events), language function (assess speech and comprehension during the interview) and general intelligence. Peripheral neuropathy is also well recognised. |
| **PERCUSSION** | This is of limited value except in confirming the size of organs or masses or in the chest for pneumonic consolidation or effusion. |
| **AUSCULTATION**<br>*Pneumonia* | A thorough examination of the chest is important to identify evidence of pneumonia. The common causes of this are likely, while pneumocystis carinii pneumonia may be present with few physical signs. |

# INDEX

Abdominal masses, 60, 62, 76, 87, 89
Abstraction, and confusion, 121
Acanthosis nigricans, 85–86
Accessory nerve, 29
Acidosis, 52, 90
Acne
  rosacea, 13, 16, 56, 86
  vulgaris, 13
Acromegaly, 3, 53, 102
  eyes in, 25
  face, 10, 11
Addison's disease, 4, 11, 12, 53
Adenoma sebaceum, 16
Adrenal tumours, 13, 62, 104
Agnosia, 111, 121
AIDS, 122, 132–134
  dementia, 134
  encephalopathy, 134
  opportunistic infections, 132, 133
  see also HIV infection
Albinism, 11
Alcohol abuse, 3, 4, 33, 57, 58, 86, 116
Alkaptonuria, 17
Alopecia, 12, 124
  frontal, 12
Alzheimer's disease, 26, 122
Amblyopia, 21
Amyloidosis, 3, 121
Amyotrophy, 67, 97
Anaemia, 4, 25, 57, 73–77, 86, 91, 124
Angioid streaks, 25
Angiomata, 57
Angular cheilitis, 15, 75
Anhydrosis, 21
Ankylosing spondylitis, 20, 40, 51, 124, 128, 129
Anomic aphasia, 112
Anosmia, 24
Antihypertensives, side effects, 105–106
Anxiety, 37
Aortic aneurysm, 35, 40, 59

Aortic dissection, 39
Aortic regurgitation, 38, 39, 40, 43, 46–47, 48, 105
Aortic sclerosis, 46
Aortic stenosis, 38, 42, 43, 46, 47, 48
Apathy, 12
Apex beat, 40, 43, 52, 104
  double, 43, 104
  tapping, 43
  thrusting, 43, 104
Aphasia, 111, 112, 120
Aphthous ulcers, 57, 133
Apraxia
  constructional, 110, 121
  dressing, 110
Arachnodactyly, 39
Arcus cornealis (senilis), 20, 38, 39
Argyll Robertson pupils, 21, 38, 115
Arrhythmias, 41
Arthritis
  mutilans, 7, 127, 129
  rashes, 125
  see also various types
Ascites, 40, 58, 64, 87, 89
Asterixis, 3, 50, 56, 87
Ataxia, 114–119
  causes, 115
  cerebellar, 114
  Friedreich's, 71, 116, 118
  gait, 108, 114
  limb, 116
  sensory, 114
  telangiectasia, 116
  truncal, 116
Ataxic nystagmus, 72
Arterio-venous malformations, 17, 48
Athlete's foot, 66
Atopic eczema, 14
Atrial fibrillation, 113
Atrial flutter, 41
Atrial septal defect, 38, 46, 47
Auditory nerves, 27–28
Auroscopy, 28

Babinski's sign, 70
Bacteriuria, 94
Baker's cyst, 39, 67
Ballottement, 62
Barrel chest, 51, 82
Basal cell carcinoma (rodent ulcer), 16
Beau's lines, 6
Behçet's syndrome, 124–131
Bell's palsy, 11, 18
Bell's sign, 27
Biliverdin, 85
Binswanger's syndrome, 123
Bladder, 62, 64, 92, 97
Blepharitis, 19
Blindness, 19
Blinking, 19, 27
Blisters, 14, 27
Blood pressure 42,49, 77, 80, 93, 97, 104–105, 122
Blue bloaters, 50
Borborygmi, 64
Bossing, frontal, 10
Bouchard's nodes, 7, 126
Bowel sounds, 64–65
Bradycardia, 40
Branchial cysts, 30
Breasts, 53, 98
    see also Gynaecomastia
Breath sounds, 54
Breathlessness, 37
Broca's aphasia, 112
Brown spots, 96
Brown-Séquard syndrome, 71–72
Brucellosis, 125
Bruising, 58, 90
Bruit
    arterial, 80, 97
    carotid, 48, 113, 123
    cranial, 123
    femoral, 48
    fistula, 93
    goitre, 36
    hepatic, 64–65, 80, 89
    renal, 93, 105
    thyroid, 36, 101
Brushfield spots, 20
Buccal mucosa, 50, 81
Budd–Chiari syndrome, 31, 32, 58, 61
Buffalo hump, 30
Bursitis, 127, 129
Butterfly rash, 124


Cachexia, 4, 10, 56, 73
Café au lait patches, 39
Calcification, corneal, 21
Calcinosis, 56, 91

Campbell de Morgan spots, 58
Candidiasis, 15, 57, 96, 133
Cannon wave, 32, 40
Capillary filling, 40
Caput medusae, 59, 87
Carbuncles, 14
Carcinoid syndrome, 12, 13
Cardiac dullness, 44, 54
Cardiac shunts, 37
Cardiomyopathy, 38, 40
Carotenaemia, 4, 12, 85
Carotico-cavernous fistula, 18, 23
Carotid stenosis, 36
Carpal tunnel syndrome, 4, 7, 127
Casts, 94
Cataracts, 21, 24, 95, 125
Cavernous sinus thrombosis, 18, 19
Cerebellum
    degeneration, 116
    haemangioblastoma, 79
Cervical rib, 4
Cervical spondylosis, 29
Cervix, 63
Chalazion, 19
Charcot's joints, 7, 96, 130
Cheeks, 10
Cheilitis, 15, 75, 76
Chemosis, 19, 99
Chest expansion, 51, 52, 83
Cheyne–Stokes respiration, 52
Chloasma, 12
Choledochal cyst, 88
Cholesterol emboli, optic fundus, 113
Chordae tendinae, rupture, 46
Chorea, 122
Chorioretinitis, 133
Choroiditis, 34
Chronic relapsing polychondritis, 16–17
Chvostek's sign, 17, 31
Cimino fistula, 91–92, 93
Circinate balanitis, 126, 129
Clasp-knife rigidity, 110, 111
Clubbing, 5, 8
    causes, 5, 38, 50, 56, 67, 74, 78, 81, 87, 100, 126
    pseudo, 5
Coarctation of aorta, 36, 46, 48, 102
Complexion, 10, 56, 85, 91
Conduction aphasia, 112
Confrontation, 22
Confusion, 120–123
    calculation problems, 121
    picture interpretation, 121
    screening tests, 120, 121
Conjunctivitis, 19
Consciousness level, 90, 95, 107, 120, 134

Constrictive pericarditis, 31–32
Continuous ambulatory peritoneal
    dialysis, 92
Cor pulmonale, 37
Cornea, 20–21, 24
    calcification, 20
    opacities, 24
    scarring, 99
    ulceration, 20
Corneal reflex, 26
Corrigan's sign, 35
Cortical sensory loss, 110
Coryza, 17
Courvoisier's law, 88
Cranial nerve palsies, 11, 18
Crepitations, 55, 83, 93, 105, 123,
    131
Crepitus, 36, 130
Creutzfeldt–Jakob disease, 122
Crico-sternal distance, 52–53
CRST syndrome, 56, 126
Cruveilhier–Baumgarten sydrome, 65
Cullen's sign, 59
Cushing's syndrome, 13, 30, 58, 67,
    102
    facies, 10, 11, 12, 86, 102, 124
Cyanosis, 37, 50, 78, 81–84
    central, 4, 81
    differential, 81
    false, 84
    peripheral, 4, 66, 81
Cytomegalovirus infection, 133

Dacryoadenitis, 19
Dactylitis, 75
Darwin's tubercle, 17
De Mussett's sign, 38
Delirium, 121
Depression, 12
Dermatitis
    contact, 10
    exfoliative, 74
    herpetiformis, 14, 58
    perioral, 13
    seborrhoeic, 13, 132
    stasis, 66
Dermatomes, legs, 71
Dermatomyositis, 6, 13, 126
Dextrocardia, 43, 54
Diabetes mellitus, 4, 14, 19, 33, 71,
    91, 95–97, 130
    eyes in, 1, 20, 24, 25
Diplopia, 22
Discoid lupus, 12
Diuretics, side effects, 105
Down's syndrome, 11, 20, 24, 38

Dresden doll face, 37
Dress sense, 121
Dressing apraxia, 110
Drowsiness, confusion, 122
Drugs
    in hypertension, 105–106
    skin rashes, 14
Dupuytren's contracture, 4, 56, 87
Duroziez's sign, 49
Dysarthria, 111
Dysdiadochokinesis, 80, 117
Dysmetria, 80, 117
Dysphagia, 29, 111
Dysphasia, 111
Dysphonia, 29
Dyspnoea, 79, 82
Dysrhythmia, 41, 100, 113
Dystrophia myotonica, 11, 12, 18, 26,
    29, 32

Ears, 17
Ecchymoses, 67, 74, 125
Ectropion, 19
Effusions, joints, 129
Ehlers–Danlos syndrome, 130
Eisenmenger's syndrome, 84
Ejection click, 45
Emotional state, 12
    agitation, 12
    apathy, 12
    euphoria, 12
    lability, 12, 121
Emphysema, 43, 50–55, 83
    subcutaneous (surgical), 33, 36
Endocarditis, infective, 8, 37, 38,
    39, 49
Enophthalmos, 21
Entropion, 19
Epilepsy, 4
Episcleritis, 20
Erysipelas, 10
Erythema
    ab igne, 125
    marginatum, 125
    multiforme, 14
    nodosum, 67, 87, 125
    palmar, 4, 56, 87, 100
Etat lacunaire, 114
Euphoria, 12
Examination technique, 1–2
Exophthalmos, 18, 19, 21, 99
Eyes, 18–25, 95–96, 99, 124–125
    conjugate deviation, 22
    deviation, 108
    glass, 19
    movements, 21–22, 95

Face, 10–17, 38, 81
  pigmented lesions, 11–12
  in strokes, 108
Facial expression, 12
  see also various diseases
Facial muscles, 27
Facial nerves, 27
Facial palsy (Bell's), 11, 18
Faeces, examination, 89
Fallot's tetralogy, 84
Fasciculation, 4, 90
  hands, 4
  legs, 68
  tongue, 29
Felty's syndrome, 131
Femoral nerve, stretch test, 71
Femoral triangle, 68
Fibrillation
  atrial, 41
  ventricular, 41
Finger–nose test, 3, 110, 117
Finger-tip atrophy, 56
Fluid thrill, 62
Flushing, 12, 13
Foetor hepaticus, 57, 86
Folliculitis, 96
Foot drop, 68, 108
Friedreich's ataxia, 71, 116, 118
Froment's sign, 8
Fundoscopy, 113, 118–119
Fundus (optic), 24, 49, 80, 91, 118
  hypertension, 91, 95, 103
Funnel chest, 39
Furuncles, 14
Gag reflex, 28, 29
Gait, 69, 70, 122
  strokes, 107
Gallbladder, 88
Gallop rhythm, 45, 83
Gangrene, 33, 66
Gas gangrene, 33
General paralysis of the insane, 29
Genitalia, 59, 88, 126
Genu valgum, 129
Gilbert's disease, 85
Gingivitis, 133
Glabellar tap, 27
Glaucoma, 21, 25
Global aphasia, 112
Globe lag, 100
Glomerulonephritis, 10, 90
Glossitis, 57, 75
Glucagonoma, 58
Goitre, 30, 33, 100–101
  retrosternal, 36, 101

Gorlin's syndrome, 16
Gout, 7, 79, 127, 128
  tophi, 7, 17, 91, 124, 127
Granny's tartan, 125
Graphaesthesia, 110
Graves' disease, 33, 99–101
Grey–Turner's sign, 59
Gums, 75–76, 133
Gynaecomastia, 53, 58, 87, 88, 101

Haemangiomas
  capillary, 16
  cavernous, 16
Haemochromatosis, 12, 57, 58
Haemodialysis, 92
Haemophilia, 125
Haemorrhoids, 63
Hair, 12–13
  body, lack of, 87
  coarsening, 13
  facial, lack of, 13
  thinning, 12–13
Halothane hepatitis, 87
Hands, 3–9, 38–39, 75, 81, 91, 100
  abnormal sensation, 8–9
  innervation, 8–9
Harrison's sulci, 39, 51
Hay fever, 17
Haygarth nodes, 7
Head nodding, 38
Hearing, 27–28
Heart, auscultation, 44–49, 101
Heart block, complete, 40
Heart failure, 4, 19, 39, 40, 43, 52, 103, 122
Heart sounds, 43, 44–45
Heberden's nodes, 7, 126
Heel–shin test, 111
Heliotrope rash, 124
Hemiplegia, 3, 103, 107, 108
  crossed, 109
Henoch–Schönlein purpura, 125
Hepatitis, B, 58, 86
Hepatojugular reflux, 31
Hepatomegaly, 43, 60, 61, 76, 79, 83, 97, 101, 121, 134
Hepatorenal syndrome, 92
Hereditary haemorrhagic telangiectasia, 57
Hernias, 59, 63
Herpes simplex, 15, 133
Herpes zoster, 15
Hess test, 74

Hiccoughs, 90
Hip, osteoarthrosis, 130
Hirsutism, 13
HIV infection, 35, 57, 86, 132–134
  classification, 133
Hoffman's sign, 110
Holmes–Adie pupil, 21
Homocystinuria, 24, 130
Hordeolum, 19
Horner's syndrome, 18, 21, 50–51
Huntington's chorea, 122
Hutchison's melanotic freckle, 16
Hydration, 95
Hygroma, cystic, 30
Hyperacusis, 27
Hypercapnia, 3, 50
Hypercholesterolaemia, 19, 39
Hyperkinesia, 99
Hypermobility, 130
Hyperphosphataemia, 25
Hyperpronation, 116
Hyperreflexia, 69, 70
Hyperresonance, 54, 83
Hypertension, 82, 93, 97, 102–106,
  108
  eyes, 25
  portal, 59
Hyperthyroidism (thyrotoxicosis), 3, 4,
  10, 12, 18, 19, 37, 99–101
  facies, 11
Hypertrophic obstructive
  cardiomyopathy, 46, 48
Hypertrophic pulmonary
  osteoarthropathy, 5, 8, 126
Hypoalbuminaemia, 39, 66, 87
Hypocalcaemia, 17
Hypoglossal nerve, 29
Hypogonadism, 13
Hypoparathyroidism, familial, nails in, 6
Hypopituitarism, 13
Hypoproteinaemia, 39
Hyporeflexia, 69
Hypotension, postural, 93
Hypothyroidism, 3, 11, 12, 19, 38, 74,
  100, 116
Hypotonia, 69
Hysteria 12,

Ileostomy, 87
Impetigo, 14
Injection marks, 86, 108, 132–133
Insulin sensitivity, 96
Intercostal indrawing, 51
Intertrigo, 96
Iridocyclitis, 34

Iris, 21
Iritis, 20
  rubeosa, 95

Janeway lesions, 58
Jaundice, 19, 56, 57, 74, 85–89, 91
Jaw jerk, 26
Joints, 7, 126–130
  active movement, 8
  examination, 128
  passive movement, 8
  tenderness, 8, 129
Jugular venous pulse, 31, 39, 40, 42,
  82, 86, 91

Kallman's syndrome, 26
Kaposi's sarcoma, 132, 133, 134
Kartagener's syndrome, 17
Kayser–Fleischer rings, 20, 56, 86
Keratitis, 20
Keratoacanthoma, 16
Keratoconjunctivitis sicca, 20
Keratoderma blenorrhagica, 67, 127,
  129
Kernig's sign, 71
Ketoacidosis, 52
Kidney
  enlarged, 76, 79, 92, 104, 121
  examination, 61–62, 131
  small, 92, 104
Kidney failure, 12
Klinefelter's syndrome, 53
Klippel–Feil syndrome, 30
Klumpke's paralysis, 4
Koilonychia, 5, 56, 74
Kussmaul's sign, 31–32
Kyphoscoliosis, 39, 51
Kyphosis, 30

Lead poisoning, 77
Left ventricular failure, 18, 37, 38
Legs, 38–39, 66–72, 79, 92, 100, 111
Lens, dislocation, 24, 38
Lentigines, 16
Lentigo maligna, 16
Leonine facies, 15
Leprosy, 15, 16
Leukaemia, 19, 25, 34, 54
Leukonychia, 5, 56, 86
Leukoplakia, hairy, 133
Lichen planus, 13
Lid lag, 18, 100
Lid retraction, 18, 100

Light eruption, polymorphic, 14
Light reflex, 21
Lindsay's nails, 5, 75, 91
Lipodystrophy, 10, 96
Lips, 81
Livedo reticularis, 125
Liver
    examination, 60, 61, 88
    failure, 3
Lown–Ganong–Levine syndrome, 41
Lupus pernio, 15
Lupus vulgaris, 15, 16
Lymph nodes, neck, 34
Lymphadenopathy, 30, 34–35, 53, 59,
        60, 76, 87–88, 134
Lymphoedema, 166
Lymphoma, 33, 34

Macula, 24
Malar flush, 12, 108
Malnutrition, 124
Marfan's syndrome, 10, 24, 38, 39,
        102, 130
Masseter, 26
Median nerve, 8
Median sternotomy, 39
Mediastinal displacement, 52
Melanin pigmentation, 11–12
Melanoma, 12, 16
Memory testing, 121
Menace reflex, 23
Meningioma, 26
Meningism, 71, 77
Menorrhagia, 77
Metastases, skin, 16
Methaemoglobinaemia, 84
Microorganisms, in urine, 94
Mikulicz's syndrome, 33–34
Milroy's disease, 66
Mitral facies, 38
Mitral regurgitation, 39, 44, 46, 47, 48
Mitral stenosis, 12, 38, 43, 44, 46, 47,
        48, 113
Mitral valve prolapse, 46, 48
Molluscum contagiosum, 15
Mononeuritis, 97
Mood, 121
Moon face, 50
    see also Cushing's disease
Motor deficit, 107
Motor neurone disease, 4, 26, 27, 29
Mucous membranes, 73, 75
Multiple endocrine adenomatosis,
        102–103
Multiple sclerosis, 12, 21, 22

Mumps, 10
Murmurs, 36, 45–48, 77, 84, 93, 105,
        113, 123, 131
    Austin Flint, 48
    Carey Coombs, 48, 131
    Graham Steel, 48
Murphy's sign, 88
Muscle
    power testing, 69, 109, 111
    tone, 68–69, 110, 111, 117–118
    wasting, 4, 67, 127, 128
Muscular dystrophy, 29
Myasthenia gravis, 18, 26, 27, 101
Myelopathy, AIDS, 134
Myocardial infarction, 37, 40
Myopathy, 67, 97, 101
Myosis, 21
Myxoedema, 3, 11, 12, 19, 38, 116
    pretibial, 67, 100

Nail bed infarcts, 6
Nail folds
    infarcts, 91, 126
    telangiectasia, 6
Nail–patella syndrome, 91
Nails, 5–6, 74, 87, 91
    absent, 6
    Beau's lines, 6
    blue lunulae, 6
    brittle, 74
    clubbing see Clubbing
    fungal infections, 6
    periungual fibroma, 6
    pitting, 6
    tar staining, 6, 78
    yellow nail syndrome, 6
Neck, 30–36, 39, 42
    webbing, 30
Necrobiosis lipoidica, 67, 96
Nephrotic syndrome, 19, 58, 92
Nerve fibres, myelinated, 25
Nerves
    cranial, 8, 26–29
    median, 8
    radial, 8
    ulnar, 8
    vagus, 28, 29
Neurofibromatosis, 4, 39, 102, 103
Neuropathy
    peripheral, AIDS, 134
    in uraemia, 92
Nikolski's sign, 14
Nodules
    rheumatic, 127
    rheumatoid, 127, 129

Nose, 16–17
  cartilage destruction, 16
  deformation, 16–17
  discharge, 17
Nystagmus, 22, 28, 116
  ataxic, 22
Obesity, 79, 107
Oedema, 3, 10, 39, 66, 74, 82, 86, 92,
    104, 129
  angioneurotic, 10
  eyelids, 19
  hand, 3
  periorbital, 19, 90–91, 104
  pulmonary, 54
Oesophagus, rupture, 33
Olecranon bursitis, 127
Onycholysis, 6, 100
Opacities, ocular, 24
Opening snap, 45
Ophthalmitis, sympathetic, 20
Ophthalmoplegia, 22, 100
Ophthalmoscopy, 21, 24
Oppenheim's test, 70
Optic atrophy, 25
Optic disc, 25
Optic neuritis, 22
Orientation testing, 121
Orthopnoea, 38
Orthosis, ankle–foot, 111
Osler's nodes, 7–8, 38
Osteoarthrosis, 7, 75, 126–131
Osteogenesis imperfecta, 20, 130


Paget's disease
  eyes, 25
  skull, 10, 11
Palatal reflex, 28
Palate, high-arched, 38
Pallor, 11, 37, 56, 66, 73
  conjunctival, 19, 56
Palms, 4
  creases, 4, 38, 73
  erythema, 4, 56, 87, 100
  hyperkeratosis, 4
Pancoast's syndrome, 51
Pancreas, 88
Papillitis, 25
Papilloedema, 25
Parasternal heave, 43
Parasternal impulse, 39
Parkinsonism
  eyes, 19, 22, 27
  face, 11, 12, 27
  tongue, 29
  tremor, 3

Parotid gland, 33–34
Parotitis, 10, 33, 57, 86
Past pointing (dysmetria), 80, 117
Patellar tap, 130
Patent ductus arteriosus, 45, 47, 48
Paterson–Brown Kelly syndrome, 57
Pectus carinatum, 39, 51, 82
Pectus excavatum, 39, 51
Pelvic tilt, 68, 129
Pelvis, examination, 77
Pemphigoid, 14
Pemphigus, 14
Percussion, 53–54
  face/head, 17
Pericardial knock, 43
Pericardial rub, 48, 93, 131
Pericarditis, 38, 40, 43, 48, 58, 93
Periodic paralysis, 101
Periorbital oedema, 19, 90, 104
Peripheral vascular disease, 66, 68, 79,
    96
Perisplenic rub, 65
Peritonitis, 59, 93
Periungual fibroma, 6
Periungual infarcts, 91
Petechiae, 74
Peutz-Jegher's syndrome, 16
Phaeochromocytoma, 18, 37, 104
Pharyngitis, 15
Pharynx, 76
Pickwickian syndrome, 79
Pigeon chest, 39, 51, 82
Pink puffers, 50
Pinna, hairy, 17
Pityriasis versicolor, 15
Plethora, 12, 78
Pleural effusions, 44
Pleural rub, 55, 83
*Pneumocystis carinii* pneumonia, 134
Poliomyelitis, 29, 67
Polyarteritis nodosa, 91
Polychondritis, relapsing, 16–17
Polycythaemia, 12, 38
  examination, 78–80
  rubra vera (primary), 78, 83
  secondary, 78, 79
  spurious, 78
Pompholyx, 4
Porphyria, 14
  cutanea tarda, 14, 57, 85
  variegata, 14
Port-wine stain, 16
Posture, 48, 68, 129
  stroke, 108
Pott's disease, spine, 51
Pregnancy, 4, 74

Pretibial myxoedema, 67, 100
Primary biliary cirrhosis, 12, 57, 85
Proctoscopy, 63
Prognathia, 10, 102
Proprioception, 97, 118
Proptosis, 18, 23, 99
Prostate, 63, 92
Protoporphyria, erythropoietic, 14
Pseudoacanthosis nigricans, 86
Pseudobulbar palsy, 12, 29
Pseudoclubbing, 5
Pseudogout, 128
Pseudohaematuria, 94
Pseudohypoparathyroidism, 7
Pseudoxanthoma elasticum, 25, 31
Psoriasis, 5, 74, 125, 127, 128
    face, 14
    nails, 6
    palms, 5
Pterygoid muscle, 26
Ptosis, 18, 21, 115
Puddle sign, 64
Pulmonary embolism, 37, 83
Pulmonary regurgitation, 47
Pulmonary stenosis, 46, 47, 48
Pulse, 40–42, 76, 82–83
    absent radial, 42
    alternans, 42
    aortic, 40
    bisferiens, 42
    bounding, 50
    capillary, 39
    carotid, 30, 35, 113
    character, 41–42
    collapsing, 42
    dicrotic, 42
    feet/peripheral, 68, 82, 96
    femoral, 63
    inequality, 42
    jerky, 42
    jugular venous, 31, 39, 40, 42, 82,
        86, 91
    paradoxus, 42
    plateau, 42
    radial, 41
    radiofemoral delay, 42, 103–104
    rhythm, 41
    volume, 42, 103
Pupils, 21–22
Purpura, 67, 125
Pyelonephritis, 92
Pyoderma gangrenosum, 58, 87

Quincke's pulse, 39

Race, anaemias, 74
Radial nerve, 8
Ramsay–Hunt syndrome, 15
Raynaud's phenomenon, 66, 126
Raynaud's syndrome, 56
Rectal examination, 63, 76, 79, 88, 92
Reflexes, 69, 70–71, 97, 122
    delayed relaxation, 118
    pendular, 70, 118
    plantar, 70, 111, 118
    stroke, 110
    tendon, 70, 110, 111
Refsum's disease, 119
Reiter's syndrome, 20, 124–131
Renal failure, 103
Respiration
    accessory muscles, 32, 51, 82
    diabetes mellitus, 95
    rate/pattern, 52
    uraemia, 90
    see also Breath sounds
Retina, 24–25, 96
Retro-orbital tumours, 19
Retrobular neuritis, 25
Rheumatoid arthritis, 47, 91, 124–131
    anaemia, 75
    boutonnière deformity, 7, 127
    eyes, 19–20
    hands, 38
    juvenile, 125, 128, 131
    swan-neck deformity, 7, 127
Rhinophyma, 16, 57, 86
Rhonchi, 54, 83, 101, 123
Rickets, 10, 39
Rickety rosary, 51
Riedel's lobe, 60
Rigidity
    clasp-knife, 110, 111
    cog-wheel, 69
    plastic, 69
Ringworm, 15
Rinne's test, 28
Rodent ulcer (basal cell carcinoma), 16
Romberg's sign, 114–115
Rossolimo's sign, 70–71
Roth spots, 49
Rubico iriditis, 20

Salivary glands, 30, 33
Sallow complexion, 56
Sarcoidosis, 10, 15, 19, 20, 33, 131
Scabies, 6
Scars, 30–31, 39, 59, 74, 87, 91, 126

Schirmer's test, 20
Sclera, 20
Sclerodactyly, 126
Scleroderma, 11, 13, 31, 38–39, 125, 128
Scleromalacia, 20, 125
Scoliosis, 51
Scratch marks, 86, 90
Scrofula, 31
Seborrhoeic dermatitis, 13, 132
Seborrhoeic keratosis, 12
Sensation
    inattention, 72, 110
    testing, 71–72, 97, 110, 111, 122
Shingles, 15
Sickle cell anaemia, 10, 75, 115
Sifting dullness, 64
Sjögren's syndrome, 20, 33, 57, 125
Skin
    diabetics, 96
    facial, 13–16
    lower limbs, 66
Skull
    enlargement, 10
    fracture, 26
Snellen chart, 23
Snout reflex, 27
Solar keratosis, 16
Spasticity, 69
Spatial disorientation, 111
Speech, 111
    rapid, 99
    scanning, 118
    staccato, 118
Spider naevi, 15, 31, 58, 87
Spinal cord
    compression, 4
    subacute combined degeneration, 77
Spleen, examination, 60–61, 88, 92–93
Splenomegaly, 61, 62, 76, 79, 83, 88, 92, 101, 122, 131, 134
Splinter haemorrhages, 6, 38, 75
Spondylosis, cervical, 4
Sputum, 52
Squamous cell carcinoma, 16, 133
Stature, 74
Stereognosis, 110
Sternomastoid tumour, 32
Sternomastoid wasting, 32
Sternum, tenderness, 54
Stevens–Johnson syndrome, 19
Stomach, carcinoma, 35
Stomatitis, 15
Stony dullness, 83
Straight back syndrome, 40, 51

Straight leg test, 71
Strawberry naevi, 16
Striae, 58
Stridor, 101
Stroke, 36, 95, 107–113, 114
    communication, 111
    coordination, 110
    movements, 108
Sturge–Weber syndrome, 16
Subacute combined degeneration, 77
Subclavian stenosis, 36
Submandibular glands, 34
Succussion splash, 63
Sulphaemoglobinaemia, 84
Supranuclear palsy, 22
Sweating, 37, 66, 95, 99, 100
Syphilis, 10, 15, 16, 19, 20, 29, 33, 34, 38
    congenital, 20
    secondary, 4, 125
Syringomyelia, 4, 7, 130
Systemic lupus erythematosus, 4, 12, 13, 14, 124, 128
Systemic sclerosis (scleroderma), 11, 13, 31, 38–39, 91, 124, 125, 126, 128

Tables dorsalis, 115, 130
Tachycardia, 83, 96
    sinus, 41, 100
    supraventricular, 41, 100
    ventricular, 41
Tachypnoea, 79, 82
Tactile vocal fremitus, 53
Takayasu's disease, 42
Taste sensation, 27
Tattoos, 58
Telangiectasia, 6, 16, 57, 75
    ataxia, 116
    herditary, haemorrhagic, 57
Temporal arteritis, 17
Terry's nails, 6
Thalamic lesions, 110
Thomas' test, 130
Thrills, 43, 113
    apical, 43
    basal, 43
    parasternal, 43
Thrombophlebitis, 68, 87
Thrush, 15, 133
Thumb finding test, 110
Thyroglossal cysts, 30
Thyroid carcinoma, 33
Thyroid hormones, 101
Thyroiditis, 33, 101

Thyrotoxicosis *see* Hyperthyroidism
Tinel's sign, 127
Titubation, 38, 116
Tongue, 27, 57, 81
Torticollis, 32
Toxic epidermal necrolysis, 14
Trachea, 52, 82, 101
 tug, 35
Trachoma, 19
Tremor
 benign essential, 3
 cerebellar, 116–117
 coarse, 3
 fine, 82, 100
 flapping, 82
 intention, 3, 117
 physiological, 3
 pill-rolling, 3
 postural, 3
 trombone, 29
Trendelenberg test , 68
Trichotillomania, 12
Tricuspid regurgitation, 31, 43, 46
Tricuspid stenosis, 48
Trigeminal nerves, 26–27
Troisier's sign, 35, 76
Trousseau's sign, 31
Tuberculosis, 19, 20, 31, 33, 34
Tuberous sclerosis, 16
 periungual fibroma, 6
Turgor, skin, 91
Turner's syndrome, 30, 102
Tylosis, 4, 56

Ulcerative colitis, 20
Ulcers
 aphthous, 57, 133
 legs, 66, 67, 96, 129
 perianal, 133
Ulnar nerve, 8
Uraemia, 3, 52, 74, 90–94
Uraemic frost, 91, 103
Urine, examination, 89, 94, 98
Uterus, fibroids, 79
Uveitis, 20, 124
Uveo-parotid syndrome, 34

Vagus nerve, 28–29

Valsalva manoeuvre, 44, 96
Varicose veins, 66, 68
Vasculitis, 67
Vena cava obstruction, 10, 32, 39,59
Venous hum
 abdominal, 65
 thoracic, 36
Venous stasis, 66, 83
Venous thrombosis, 39, 67, 68, 79,
 82, 108
Ventricular ectopics, 41
Ventricular heave, 83, 104
Ventricular hypertrophy, 39
Ventricular septal defect, 43, 46, 47
Vertigo, 22
Vibration, 71–72, 79
Vincent's angina, 76
Virchow's node, 35, 75
Visual acuity, 23, 95
Visual fields, 22, 23
Vitamin $B_{12}$ deficiency, 71, 73
Vitiligo, 11, 31, 85, 99, 115
Vocal resonance, 53, 55
von Hippel–Lindau syndrome, 102

Warts, 15
 perianal, 133
Weber's test, 28
Wegener's granulomatosis, 16
Weight loss, 86, 99
Weil's disease, 91, 92
Wernicke's aphasia, 112
Wernicke's encephalopathy, 4
Wharton's duct obstruction, 34
Wheezes, 54, 83, 101, 123
Whipple's disease, 126
Whispering pectoriloquy, 54
Wilson's disease
 eyes, 20, 56, 86
 nails, 6
Wolff–Parkinson–White syndrome, 41

Xanthelasma, 16, 19, 39, 56, 86
Xanthomas, 39
Xerostomia, 34, 125